ATLAS OF
TRANSVAGINAL
SURGERY

ATLAS OF
TRANSVAGINAL
SURGERY

Shlomo Raz, M.D.

Division of Urology

University of California

School of Medicine

Los Angeles, California

W.B. SAUNDERS

A Division of Harcourt Brace & Company

Philadelphia London Toronto Montreal Sydney Tokyo

W.B. SAUNDERS COMPANY
A Division of
Harcourt Brace & Company

The Curtis Center
Independence Square West
Philadelphia, Pennsylvania 19106

Library of Congress Cataloging-in-Publication Data

Raz, Shlomo,

    Atlas of transvaginal surgery / Shlomo Raz.
      p.   cm.
    Includes index.

    ISBN 0-7216-2431-6

    I. Vagina—Surgery—Atlases.   I. Title.
    |DNLM: I. Vagina—surgery—atlases. 2. Vaginal Diseases—surgery—
      atlases.   WP 17 R278a|

RG104.R38   1992
618.1'5059'0222—dc20

DNLM/DLC   92-3581

Editor: W. B. Saunders Staff
Designer: Paul Fry
Production Manager: Peter Faber
Manuscript Editor: Wynette Kommer
Illustration Specialist: Brett MacNaughton
Page Layout Artist: W. B. Saunders Staff
Indexer: Helene Taylor

Atlas of Transvaginal Surgery   ISBN 0-7216-2431-6

Printed in the United States of America.

9   8   7   6   5   4   3

DEDICATION

To my wife

Sylvia

and my children

Alan, Yael, Daniela and **Karyn**

For their love and support.

FOREWORD

Over the past 20 years, Shlomo Raz and I have been interested in the same areas of clinical medicine and surgery. During that time, both of us modified our concepts regarding the pathophysiology of the conditions we encountered, our methods of diagnosis, and our surgical management of these conditions, in a painful process of evolution. In passing, I learned more from Shlomo than he ever learned from me. This work is a professional distillation of a lifetime of work by a surgeon who concentrated on the development of a comprehensive, reality-based, surgical discipline. The changes that have occurred in the area of female urology in the past 15 years are revolutionary, and Dr. Raz has been largely responsible for those changes. Without suffering the inevitable false passages, the painful revisions of long-held concepts, and the abandonment of cherished ideas that turned out to be incorrect, the reader can enjoy the end product of the work of one of the most innovative, intellectually curious, and tireless surgeons of our time. There is no other work like this one. Everything is here—all the nuances in technique and all the lessons and skills taught by experience. It is my great privilege to be a part of it. These techniques apply to both urology and for gynecology and represent a solid step forward for the patients we treat.

EDWARD J. McGUIRE, M.D.

INTRODUCTION

It is indeed strange that after completing all the chapters of this atlas, I must come back and write the beginning. This atlas is not intended to cover all vaginal operations but rather is limited to the most common reconstructive procedures. No procedures for atypia, cancer, stones, and abnormal uterine bleeding are included. The scope of this atlas is also limited because it does not include all available surgical techniques for the diverse conditions. Instead, it reflects my *personal* approach to vaginal reconstructive surgery. Some of the procedures that will be described were inspired or modified from other techniques but, for better or for worse, this is the way I do them.

A better understanding of the anatomy and physiology of bladder function and support led to the development of newer and effective techniques to correct vaginal prolapse and urinary incontinence. The chapter on the anatomy of continence and pelvic support covers some of the aspects of our new understanding of bladder and pelvic support, urethral physiology, and diagnosis that led to the development of these new procedures.

Female genitourinary surgery has evolved dramatically in recent years, particularly in the field of vaginal operations for incontinence. For more than 70 years the main operation for urinary incontinence and cystocele was any modification of the Kelly plication. Now it is a general consensus that anterior colporraphy should be abandoned in the treatment of urinary incontinence. Urinary stress incontinence is divided into two main groups: anatomic and intrinsic sphincter dysfunction. In patients with anatomic incontinence (AI), the sphincteric unit is intact but malpositioned. The goal of operation for anatomic incontinence is repositioning of the bladder neck and urethra to a high retropubic position. Patients with intrinsic sphincter dysfunction (ISD) have a sphincteric unit damaged by a neurologic condition (myelomeningocele, sacral arc lesion), pelvic trauma, radiation, or multiple operations. The goal of surgery for ISD is to provide compression, support, and coaptation to the sphincteric unit. Bladder neck suspension procedures are generally not effective in these cases, so other alternatives, such as slings and periurethral bulking procedures, are to be considered. Patients with ISD constitute almost 10 percent of our very selective practice. The vaginal wall and fascial sling procedures, as well as the use of Teflon injections for ISD, are described in detail.

In patients with anatomic incontinence, the degree of anterior vaginal wall prolapse usually dictates the type of operation required to correct urinary incontinence. Patients with stress incontinence who have minimal urethral and bladder hypermobility are generally cured by a bladder neck suspension. Patients with significant cystourethrocele with or without stress incontinence require not only a suspension procedure for the urethral and bladder neck but also an operation to correct bladder prolapse. Cystocele may be the result of a central defect (weakness between the two pubocervical fasciae), with preservation of the lateral bladder support, or may be due to a sliding herniation of the lateral, paravaginal support. We have included our technique of cystocele repair in patients with significant grade IV cystocele, in which we provide elevation of the bladder neck, repair of the central defect, and support of the bladder and urethra in a high retropubic position. Selected patients with lateral (paravaginal) cystocele can be treated without repairing the hernia defect but rather by support and elevation of the bladder base and bladder neck by a simpler technique such as the four corner bladder and bladder neck suspension.

Urinary incontinence is rarely an isolated condition; generally it is simply a manifestation of pelvic floor relaxation. Focusing attention on the treatment of urinary incontinence and urethral hypermobility without simultaneous treatment of significant rectocele, enterocele, or uterine prolapse is a mistake. The chapters on rectocele and enterocele repair, vaginal hysterectomy for prolapse, and sacrospinalis fixation for vaginal vault prolapse cover the approach to this particular problem.

Vaginal reconstructive surgery should be in the hands of surgeons with the expertise to understand, diagnose, and perform vaginal surgery. This craft should include also the diagnosis and treatment of any complications that may derive from vaginal reconstructive surgery. Proper surgical training and knowledge of voiding dysfunction, urodynamics, cystoscopy, endourology, ureteric catheterization, stent insertion, bowel reconstruction, and other such procedures are imperative when vaginal operations are contemplated. Complications of surgery are discussed with each of the surgical procedures, and also a general chapter on complications of vaginal operations is included.

Vesicovaginal fistula is one of the most important complications of hysterectomy, pelvic radiation, and other pelvic procedures. Important and controversial issues always arise within its treatment. The timing of surgery (whether early or late), the vaginal or abdominal approach, and use of adjunctive procedures like Martius flaps and vaginal flaps are discussed. The best operation for fistula is the first, and the first operation should be the one with which the surgeon is most familiar. Using sound surgical principles and proper exposure and dissection, as well as the proper use of adjunctive procedures, makes the vaginal approach our procedure of choice for the majority of fistula repairs. The vaginal approach offers the advantages of minimal morbidity, shorter hospital stay, and equally good results.

Recurrent urinary tract infections are very common in women. Although the majority of patients will respond to conservative measures and further testing is not revealing, a small group of patients will suffer from urethral diverticula as the source of the infection. We describe our technique of excision of urethral diverticula that is indicated in the very symptomatic patient with mid or proximal urethral diverticula.

Absent vagina may be congenital or due to surgical excision during cancer surgery. Construction of a neovagina using skin graft, myocutaneous flaps, and bowel is presented. The urethra may be extensively damaged by trauma, surgery, radiation, or delivery. Under construction of neourethra, we discuss this challenging operation. In this case the aim of operation is to restore continence and to reconstruct the urethral canal for normal transport of urine outside the vagina. In more extensive cases in which the urethra is totally destroyed, reconstruction is not desired. We present our technique of transvaginal closure of the bladder neck. This procedure can be performed by itself or as part of a more comprehensive reconstruction, such as cystoplasty and construction of a continent nipple for self-catheterization.

In the majority of the chapters, the reader will find a simple format: indications, diagnosis, surgical technique, and intraoperative and late complications. Diagrams complement intraoperative photographs for each of the surgical steps. No suggested literature or extensive surgical descriptions are provided because the pictures speak for themselves. This atlas would not be possible without the invaluable help of Gwynne Gloege, medical illustrator of the Department of Surgery at the UCLA School of Medicine. With great dedication and superb expertise, she was able to transform my operative descriptions into clear diagrams that provide the impact and dimension needed to clarify the different surgical steps.

CONTENTS

THE ANATOMY OF PELVIC SUPPORT AND STRESS INCONTINENCE

Clinical, urodynamic, radiologic, and endoscopic evaluations, as well as operative experience on over 800 cases of stress incontinence, have led us to a better understanding of the pathophysiology of female stress incontinence. We will correlate those concepts with anatomic dissections obtained from whole mount and step sections of the female pelvis as well as with magnetic resonance images of the female pelvis, the paraurethral and bladder neck area in patients with known stress incontinence, and normal control women. Our findings support a simplified conceptual understanding of the anatomy of stress incontinence, allowing more rational treatment of this common disorder.

Stress urinary incontinence, or the involuntary loss of urine through the intact urethra as a result of a sudden increase in intra-abdominal pressure, which is a social problem to the patient, is the end-result of a deficient urinary control system. Failure of this system results in intra-abdominal pressure exceeding the resistance produced by the urethral closure mechanisms. Normal continence in women results from the delicate balance of several forces, including closing pressure of the urethra, a critical functional and anatomic urethral length, the ability of the pelvic floor to increase urethral pressure at the time of stress, and the proper anatomic location of the sphincteric unit. Normally, anatomic support of the bladder neck and proximal urethra allows for through transmission of intra-abdominal pressure increases to this area that controls continence. Through an intrinsically intact urethra with its coapting mucosal surface and the reflex pelvic contraction at the time of cough or strain, a leak-proof sphincter is achieved.

Failure of one of the components of this delicate balance does not invariably produce stress incontinence, because of the compensatory effect of other factors. This may explain why patients with a very short urethra (such as after distal excision or incision) are continent if the bladder neck and urethra are in good anatomic position and the remaining urethra preserves good closing pressures. On the other hand, if this short urethra is hypermobile and prolapsed, incontinence will occur. This also may explain the phenomenon in which many patients with urethral and bladder prolapse can be totally asymptomatic.

Obstetric trauma and the resulting anatomic displacements occur between the ages of 20 and 30 years, but "anatomic incontinence" is found mainly around the menopause, suggesting that hormonal changes, such as atrophy of urethral tissue, are superimposed on the anatomic defect, producing the resultant leakage. Stress incontinence, therefore, seems to occur as a result of failure of compensatory mechanisms when one factor such as anatomy is abnormal.

There is no doubt that the underlying anatomy is of great importance in urinary stress incontinence. It is, however, important to remember that anatomic defects are but one factor in a complex mechanism of pelvic floor relaxation. The actual anatomic basis of these pathophysiologic concepts is an area of both confusion and controversy, yet it is only through a clear conceptual understanding of the anatomy involved that rational treatment can be given.

ANATOMY OF PELVIC SUPPORT

The bony pelvis is the framework upon which all pelvic structures ultimately depend. If the pelvic bone is the scaffolding, the pelvic diaphragm and perineal musculature that attach to this scaffolding provide the floor upon which the pelvic organs rest.

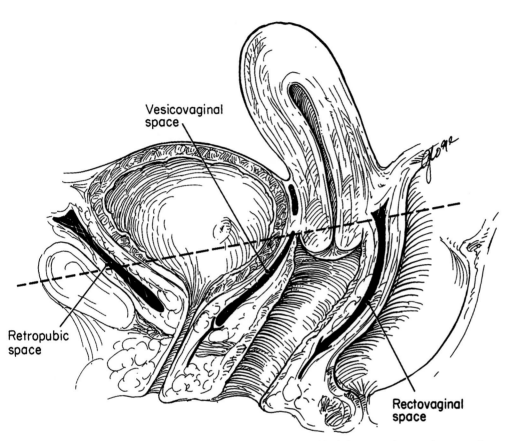

FIGURE 1–1. Lateral view of the pelvic structures, highlighting in black the surgical spaces important in vaginal surgery. The retropubic space, between bladder and pubic bone, is entered during bladder neck suspensions. The vesicovaginal space, between bladder and vaginal wall, is used at the time of formal cystocele repair to dissect free the anterior vaginal wall. At the level of the bladder neck and urethra, the perivaginal fasciae and periurethral fasciae are fused. The rectovaginal space, between the vagina and rectum, is penetrated during rectocele repair. In the distal half of the vagina, the prerectal fasciae and perivaginal fasciae are fused.

A VAGINAL VIEW

FIGURE 1–2. The retropubic, vesicovaginal and rectovaginal spaces are seen at the level of the cervix. The cardinal and sacrouterine ligaments provide support to the cervix and indirectly to the bladder base.

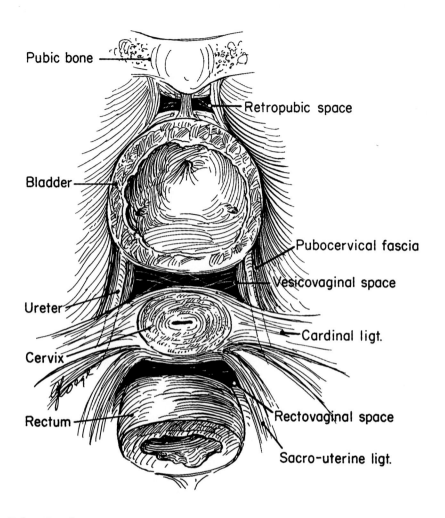

Pubic bone

Retropubic space

Bladder

Pubocervical fascia

Vesicovaginal space

Ureter

Cardinal ligt.

Cervix

Rectum

Rectovaginal space

Sacro-uterine ligt.

Pelvic Diaphragm

The pelvic diaphragm can be divided into the levator ani and coccygeus muscles. The levator ani with its component parts, the pubococcygeus, iliococcygeus, and ischiococcygeus muscles, can be viewed as the major inferior support of the urethra, vagina, and rectum. Standard anatomy texts describe the levator muscle together with its surrounding fascia as a broad, thin sheet extending from the pelvic portion of the pubic bone lateral to the symphysis anteriorly and to the inner surface of the ischial spine posteriorly. Between these points it originates by the so-called "arcuate line" of the obturator fascia (tendinous arc). From these origins the fibers extend back medially to unite with the fibers from the opposite side. In its anterior portion, the levator muscle forms a U-shaped hiatus through which the vagina, rectum, and urethra exit from the abdominal cavity (Figs. 1–2, 1–3). Fibers of the pubococcygeus muscle send a number of muscle fingers into this U-shaped hiatus. Around the urethra they form its external sphincter. The fibers fuse laterally and anteriorly to the rectum, forming part of the perineal support. The proximal half of the vagina lies horizontally over the levator plate.

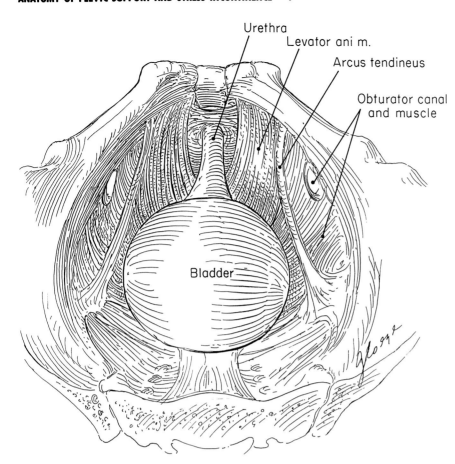

Urethra
Levator ani m.
Arcus tendineus
Obturator canal and muscle
Bladder

FIGURE 1–3. Abdominal view of the pelvic anatomy. The levator and coccygeus muscles support the pelvic viscera. The medial edges of the levator muscles fuse posteriorly, but anteriorly they form a hiatus for the passage of the urethra, vagina, and rectum. The pubococcygeal segment of the levator complex originates in the tendinous arc, a thickening of the obturator fascia. (From Walsh PC, Gittes RF, Perlmutter AD, Stamey TA: Campbell's Urology, 6th ed. Philadelphia, WB Saunders, 1992.)

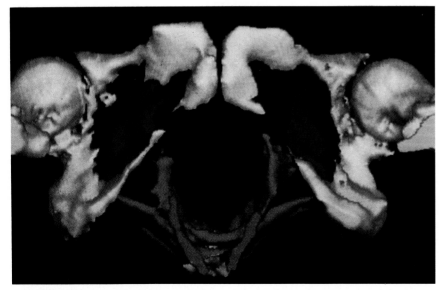

FIGURE 1–4. Three-dimensional magnetic resonance image reconstruction of the levator musculature (in green), the bony pelvis (in white), and the obturator musculature (in red). In the normal patient, the levator hiatus is wide. The rectum, vagina, and urethrovesical unit cross this hiatus, obtaining support from the levator fascia with its different condensations.

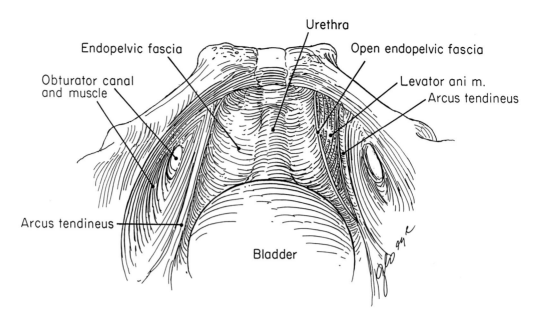

FIGURE 1–5. The pelvic viscera are covered by the endopelvic fascia. At the bladder neck and urethral level two areas of specialization are found: (1) the pubourethral ligaments attach the midurethral area to the inferior rami of the symphysis pubis; and (2) the urethropelvic ligament anchors the urethra and bladder neck to the tendinous arc. It is formed by a fusion of periurethral and endopelvic fasciae. In the right side the urethropelvic ligament is detached from the tendinous arc, as in a Raz bladder neck suspension. (From Walsh PC, Gittes RF, Perlmutter AD, Stamey TA: Campbell's Urology, 6th ed. Philadelphia, WB Saunders, 1992.)

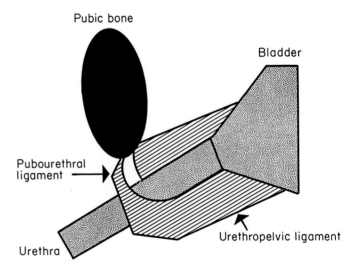

FIGURE 1–6. Diagram of urethral support. The urethropelvic ligament attaches to the tendinous arch (obturator fascia) and the pubourethral ligament to the inferior rami of the symphysis. Both these ligaments are not individual structures but rather they are specialized segments of the same fascial supporting unit. The pubourethral ligament divides the urethra into two segments: the proximal half, intra-abdominal, responsible for passive continence, and the distal half, extra-abdominal, responsible for active continence. The midurethral area (insertion of this ligament with the skeletal musculature located just distal to it) corresponds to the high-pressure zone of urethral profilometry and the area of active continence (voluntary and reflex). (From Walsh PC, Gittes RF, Perlmutter AD, Stamey TA: Campbell's Urology, 6th ed. Philadelphia, WB Saunders, 1992.)

Thus, the levator ani holds the intrapelvic organs like a hammock, providing support as well as stabilization during increases in intra-abdominal pressure. Further dissection of this muscle, however, indicates a more complex anatomy than this simple description would suggest. In comparison with other skeletal muscles of the body, the levator muscle has a much greater connective tissue make-up, and fibers arising anteriorly condense into tough bands engaging in support of the pelvic viscera directly. The fascial layer covering the levator muscle (endopelvic fascia, Fig. 1–4) at the level of the urethra and bladder neck has several distinct areas of specialization: the pubourethral, urethropelvic, the vesicopelvic (pubocervical) and cardinal ligaments. (Fig. 1–5).

Pubourethral Ligaments

The pubourethral ligaments are the best described. They connect the inner surface of the pubic bone with the midurethra. They help support and stabilize the urethra and anterior vaginal wall to the inferior aspect of the pubic bone. Weakness in these ligaments permits posterior and inferior movement of the midurethra but does not contribute significant support to the bladder neck. Just distal to these ligaments, the skeletal muscle fibers (external sphincter of the urethra) are located.

The pubourethral ligaments divide the urethra into two halves (Fig. 1–6). The proximal half, intra-abdominal, is responsible for passive continence and the distal half, extra-abdominal, is responsible for active continence (Fig. 1–6).

If one now examines the anterior vagina after an incision is made in the midline and the vaginal wall is reflected laterally (Fig. 1–7), one encounters a distinctive anatomy.

We will describe the structures responsible for urethral, bladder, and uterine support: (1) urethropelvic ligament, (2) pubocervical fascia, and (3) cardinal ligaments.

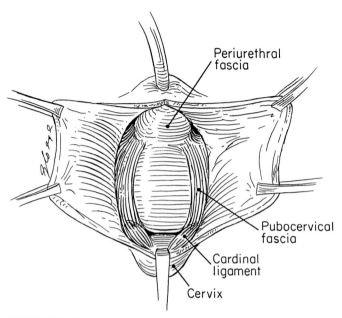

FIGURE 1–7. Vaginal view of the supporting rectangle of the anterior vaginal wall. The periurethral fascia forms the superior side of the rectangle. Covering the urethra and bladder neck, it extends beneath the pubic bone, fuses with the endopelvic fascia to form the urethropelvic ligament, and attaches to the fascia of the obturator muscle (tendinous arc). The pubocervical fascia extends laterally, supporting the bladder base with the levator muscle. The base of the rectangle is formed by the cardinal ligaments as they attach to the cervix in the midline. (From Walsh PC, Gittes RF, Perlmutter AD, Stamey TA: Campbell's Urology, 6th ed. Philadelphia, WB Saunders, 1992.)

Urethropelvic Ligaments

Another specialized group of fibers of greater functional significance to stress incontinence is the musculofascial attachments of the urethra and bladder neck to the lateral pelvic wall. The endopelvic fascia is fused to the periurethral fascia and supports like two wings the urethra to the tendinous arc, the line of insertion of the levator muscles on the obturator fascia. We have named this fascial complex the urethropelvic ligament, and it is the major support of the bladder neck and proximal urethra.

It is important to realize that the pubourethral and urethropelvic ligaments are not separate structures but merely discrete condensations of the levator fascial sheet as it attaches to the urethra and bladder neck. As will be described later, it is the urethropelvic ligament that is most important in surgical cure of anatomic stress incontinence, for it is ultimately responsible for bladder neck support.

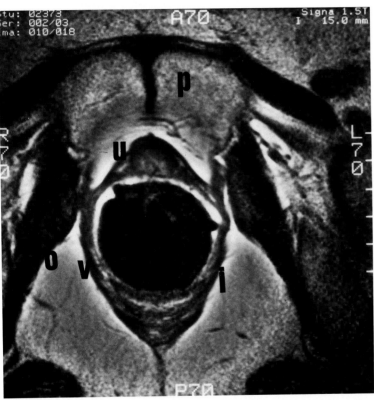

FIGURE 1–8. Magnetic resonance imaging of the urethropelvic ligament. The vagina (in black) is round and distended by an intravaginal coil. The urethropelvic ligament is seen stretching from the urethra to the tendinous arc (insertion site of the levator muscle to the obturator fascia). p, pubic bone, u, urethra, v, vaginal wall distended by coil, o, obturator muscle, and l, levator muscle.

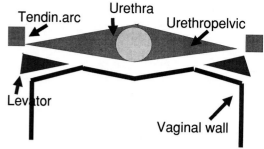

FIGURE 1–9. The urethropelvic ligament has two components: an abdominal side (the endopelvic fascia) and a vaginal side, the periurethral fascia. The levator muscle does not support directly the urethra and bladder neck but supports them indirectly by its close relation with the urethropelvic ligament. During transvaginal surgery and periurethral dissection, the medial edge of the levator hiatus is found anterior to the urethropelvic ligament. (From Walsh PC, Gittes RF, Perlmutter AD, Stamey TA: Campbell's Urology, 6th ed. Philadelphia, WB Saunders, 1992.)

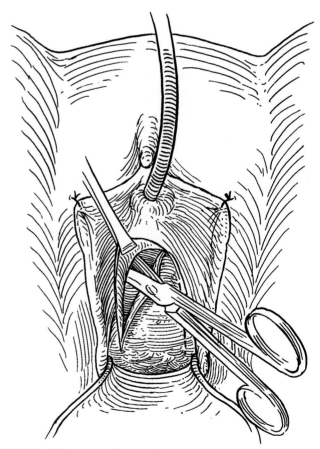

FIGURE 1–10. Diagram showing dissection of the vaginal wall over the periurethral fascia.

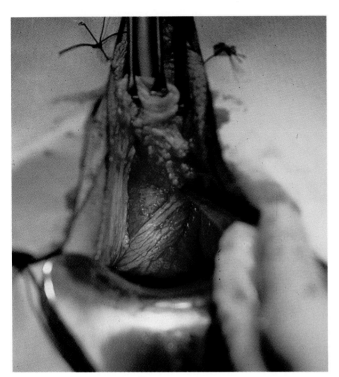

FIGURE 1–11. Photograph showing how the lateral and superficial dissection of the vaginal wall exposes the glistening periurethral fascia as it fuses with the endopelvic fascia to form the urethropelvic ligament.

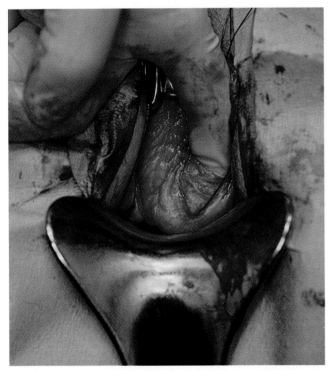

FIGURE 1–12. Further dissection around the periurethral fascia toward its insertion into the obturator fascia allows entrance into the retropubic space and exposure of the urethropelvic ligament. It is defined as the complex of fibrous structures supporting the urethra and bladder neck to the lateral pelvic wall, conceptually a fusion of the periurethral and endopelvic fasciae.

URETHRAL SUPPORT

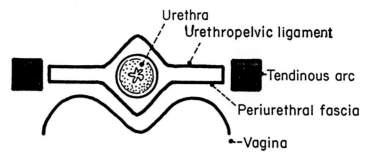

FIGURE 1—13. The periurethral and endopelvic fasciae (urethropelvic ligament) support the urethra and bladder neck like two wings against the lateral pelvic wall. These fasciae enclose the urethral wall, providing elastic support. Increased tension of this ligament by contraction of the levator or obturator muscle will increase coaptation of the urethral wall. (From Walsh PC, Gittes RF, Perlmutter AD, Stamey TA: Campbell's Urology, 6th ed. Philadelphia, WB Saunders, 1992.)

Dissection of the periurethral fascia is avascular, but there is a loose attachment to the vaginal wall that can be easily separated. No distinct plane or space is encountered; instead, the vagina and urethra are lightly fused so that the vaginal wall conforms to the shape of this periurethral fascia and follows its anatomy (Fig. 1–13). In a normal woman, the vaginal wall ascends laterally and superiorly and attaches loosely to the urethropelvic fascia in its anchor to the lateral pelvic floor, thereby giving the characteristic H shape of cross-sectional imaging of the vaginal lumen.

The periurethral fascia can be considered as the vaginal side of the urethropelvic ligament covering the intrinsic sphincteric unit. Just lateral to the urethra, it fuses with the endopelvic fascia (the abdominal component of the urethropelvic ligament), and both insert in the tendinous arc. They provide strong and elastic support of the bladder neck and urethra attaching to the lateral pelvic wall. Contraction of the levator or obturator muscles will increase the tensile forces of the urethropelvic ligaments, improving seal and continence. Weakness of the levator plate and the urethropelvic ligaments will produce urethral and bladder neck hypermobility, reducing the efficiency of the proximal urethra (Fig. 1–14).

URETHRAL PROLAPSE

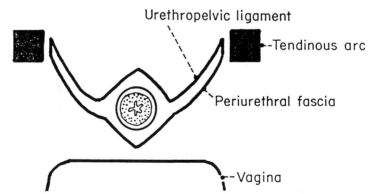

FIGURE 1—14. Multiple deliveries and estrogenic deficit contribute to the attenuation and relaxation of the levator plate and the urethropelvic ligaments. The sphincteric unit is moved to a poorly supported, dependent position, and anatomic incontinence may occur. Contraction of the levators or obturators will not increase the tension of the urethropelvic ligaments, and the coaptation of the urethral wall will be impaired.

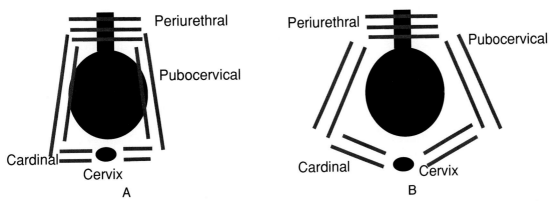

FIGURE 1–15. A, Diagram of the normal supporting rectangle of the bladder with its sides formed by the periurethral, pubocervical, and cardinal ligaments. B, In patients with pelvic floor relaxation and significant cystocele, the normal supporting rectangle of the bladder is affected. The cardinal ligaments are lax, the uterus is hypermobile, and the pubocervical fascia is attenuated and laterally displaced, facilitating the central herniation of the bladder. The goal of cystocele repair includes bladder suspension and repair of the defective rectangle by approximation of the pubocervical fascia and cardinal ligaments. (From Walsh PC, Gittes RF, Perlmutter AD, Stamey TA: Campbell's Urology, 6th ed. Philadelphia, WB Saunders, 1992.)

Pubocervical Fascia (Vesicopelvic Ligament)

When lateral dissection of the vagina is carried out at the level of the bladder, one encounters the pubocervical fascia just beneath the vaginal wall (see Fig. 1–7).

This fascia supports the bladder to the lateral pelvic wall (tendinous arc and levator muscle) (Fig. 1–15). We prefer to use the term vesicopelvic ligaments to include the fascial support of the bladder to the lateral pelvic wall. Like the urethropelvic ligament, the vesicopelvic ligament has an abdominal side (endopelvic) and a vaginal side (pubocervical fascia). The trauma of delivery, hormonal deficiency, and pelvic floor relaxation may produce three types of abnormalities of bladder support: a central defect, a lateral defect (paravaginal), or a combination of both, which is the most common finding. In patients with a central defect, the bladder is herniated in the midline, through the attenuated pubocervical fascia, while the lateral support of the bladder is preserved. In patients with lateral defects, the attachment of the bladder to the lateral pelvic wall is defective, resulting in a sliding hernia of the bladder and pubocervical fascia.

Cardinal Ligaments

The cardinal ligaments are described in more detail here not only because of their importance to uterine support, but also because of their significant impact on bladder support, incontinence, bladder prolapse, and vaginal reconstructive surgery (see Fig. 1–2). The cardinal ligaments extend from the uterine isthmus to the lateral pelvic wall (obturator and levator fasciae). The ligaments are thick and triangular and contain the uterine arteries. Posteriorly, they are fused with the sacrouterine ligaments. Superiorly, they merge with the endopelvic fascia (covering bladder and vagina). The anterior extensions of the cardinal ligaments fuse with the pubocervical fascia. The periurethral and pubocervical fasciae and cardinal ligaments form the base of a rectangle that is responsible for bladder support. Relaxation of the cardinal ligaments (as in uterine prolapse or after hysterectomy) will widen the base of the rectangle, separating its sides (the pubocervicals), and will open a wide gap into which the bladder can herniate (Fig. 1–15). We will discuss later the repair of Grade IV cystocele and the importance of repositioning the cardinal ligaments and their approximation to the midline.

CLINICAL CORRELATES

We can now make a clinical correlation between the different anatomic defects of the anterior vaginal wall. We must emphasize the importance of the insertion of the urethropelvic ligament into the lateral pelvic wall (tendinous arc and obturator fascia). The urethra is seen to be suspended from the lateral pelvic wall and enclosed like a sandwich between the vaginal and urethral side of the levator fascia. This fascial extension provides both strength and elasticity to the urethral support so as to rise and fall with changes in intra-abdominal pressure.

The pubourethral ligaments divide the urethra into two areas of continence. The distal half is responsible for active continence. The proximal half is intrapelvic, intra-abdominal, and responsible for passive continence. The area just distal to the pubourethral ligaments is outside the realm of the intra-abdominal forces; it is covered by the extension of the levator muscles and is the area of ''high pressure'' when urethral pressure studies are performed.

Passive continence (resting involuntary control) is provided by the integrity, coaptation, and support of the proximal half of the urethra. The spongy tissue surrounded by a thin musculofascial layer creates an effective seal. The tensile force of the urethropelvic ligaments surrounding the urethra and indirectly the levator musculature provides further coaptation to the proximal urethra. But other factors are also important. A true valvular effect is created by the high retropubic fixation of the bladder neck, with the bladder base being in the most dependent position. The midurethral area, through the basic tone of the skeletal musculature, provides further compression (pressure) of the spongy urethra.

In the normal continent patient, during any stress like coughing, straining, or walking a complex compensatory mechanism is ready to improve the seal effect of the urethra. Sudden changes in abdominal pressure elicit a reflex contraction of the levator muscle and an increase of midurethral pressure. Posterior bladder rotation against a well-supported urethra will increase the valvular effect of the bladder neck. Voluntary or reflex contraction of the levator and obturator muscles increases tension on the urethropelvic ligament, thereby elevating and compressing the proximal urethra. Direct transmission of intra-abdominal forces to the well-supported proximal urethra increases its closing mechanism.

Pelvic floor relaxation and weakening of the urethropelvic and pubourethral ligaments leads to posterior and downward rotation of the proximal urethra and bladder neck. The compensatory mechanism and improved seal of the proximal urethra against sudden changes in abdominal pressures are lost.

Urethral hypermobility will transfer the bladder neck area to a dependent position in the pelvis, where sudden increases in intra-abdominal pressures will facilitate its funneling and opening. The valvular effect is lost. A weak levator will not increase midurethral pressures efficiently. The urethropelvic ligaments are stretched and weak, diminishing the increase in coaptation of the proximal urethra during stress. The intra-abdominal forces are not transmitted efficiently to the proximal urethra because of loss of the supporting backboard effect of the normal strong support of the levator muscles and urethropelvic ligaments.

Surgical transfer of the proximal urethra to a high, supported position will restore some of the urethral compensatory mechanisms against sudden changes in abdominal pressure. The bladder neck is moved away from this disadvantaged position to a more protected one, where the bladder base will be in the most dependent location and a valvular effect will prevail.

Bladder neck and urethral fixation restore the supporting backboard effect needed for efficient transmission of intra-abdominal forces. Restoring tension on the urethropelvic ligaments improves the seal effect of the proximal urethra; however, an increase in midurethral pressure during coughing is probably not restored.

Surgical Correlates

Armed with this better understanding of the anatomy of stress incontinence, what surgical correlates can be drawn? First, with a conceptual picture of the structures involved in support of the bladder neck and proximal urethra, the clinician gains a better understanding of what occurs when surgical therapy is employed. The various types of bladder neck suspensions all attempt to reposition the bladder neck and proximal urethra into a high, fixed retropubic position. As one gains a better view of the supporting structures, it becomes clear that what structures are resuspended and, perhaps more important, where they are grasped have an impact on the eventual outcome. When the supporting fascia is grasped too close to the urethra, obstruction and iatrogenic damage are a danger. When it is grasped too distal to the bladder neck and proximal urethra, insufficient suspension of the continence mechanism occurs, and no improvement in symptoms will be achieved.

Patients with stress incontinence and minimal cystocele in general have hypermobility of the bladder neck and urethra because of an attenuated levator plate and urethropelvic ligaments. Patients with moderate cystocele have a similar defect, in conjunction with attenuation of the pubocervical fascia. Patients with severe anterior vaginal prolapse have a combination of anatomic abnormalities that include urethral hypermobility due to attenuated urethropelvic ligament and cystocele due to weak cardinal ligaments and pubocervical fascia (lateral and/or central defects).

In cases of bladder neck and urethral hypermobility alone, corrective surgery should restore the normal anatomy by creating a strong anchor of the urethropelvic ligaments and vaginal wall.

In patients with severe cystocele, the supporting rectangle of the bladder (the base formed by the cardinal ligaments, the sides by the pubocervical fascia, and the top by the periurethral fascia) is damaged. Two defects may be found and should be repaired accordingly: (1) The central defect of the rectangle should be repaired by medial approximation of the laterally retracted cardinals and pubocervical fascia and (2) the downward, sliding herniation of the whole bladder (paravaginal hernia) should be repaired by suspension and support of the bladder. This can be accomplished by an abdominal approach like the Burch or paravaginal colposuspension. In Chapter 5 we describe a transvaginal approach using a bladder neck and bladder suspension technique, in which permanent sutures suspend the cardinal ligaments, the pubocervical fascia, and bladder neck to the pubic bone without the need to open the abdomen.

In patients with moderate cystocele, the classic approach has been similar to that of repair of a large cystocele. Nevertheless in selected cases with mainly lateral (paravaginal) herniation of the bladder, we perform a transvaginal suspension of the bladder neck (urethropelvic ligaments) and bladder base (pubocervical and cardinal complex). We call this operation a four corner bladder neck and bladder suspension.

Later in this atlas will be found an in-depth review of the various types of surgery for anatomic incontinence. However, in Figures 1–16, 1–17, and 1–18 the more commonly used transvaginal and abdominal suspensions are illustrated as they relate to the underlying supporting structures. In the Burch suspension, the sutures include the vaginal wall and urethropelvic ligament far laterally to the urethra, anchoring them to Cooper's ligament. The Marshall-Marchetti procedure applies sutures to the urethropelvic fascia in close proximity to the urethra. The Stamey suspension relies upon suspending sutures and a vascular graft bolster applied to the inferior aspect of this fascia, in close proximity to the bladder neck. The Gittes suspension includes sutures only of the vaginal wall transferred through the urethropelvic ligament. The Raz bladder neck suspension breaks the lateral attachment of the urethropelvic fascia to provide mobility of the anterior vaginal wall and the medial edge of the open fascia. The anchoring sutures include the vaginal wall and the urethropelvic and pubocervical fasciae as laterally as possible, to achieve support without interference with the intrinsic urethral mechanism.

ABDOMINAL SUSPENSIONS

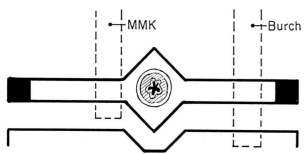

FIGURE 1–16. The Marshall-Marchetti operation includes sutures of the urethropelvic ligament in close proximity to the urethral wall, whereas the Burch type of suspension includes the vaginal wall and urethropelvic ligament far laterally diminishing the chances of obstruction.

ANTERIOR REPAIR

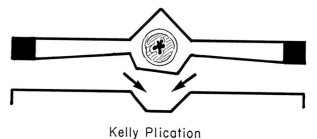

Kelly Plication

FIGURE 1–17. Anterior colporrhaphy (Kelly's operation) plicates the periurethral fascia in an attempt to improve support and coaptation of the urethral wall.

TRANSVAGINAL SUSPENSIONS

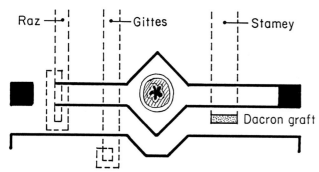

FIGURE 1–18. The Stamey type of suspension includes the use of a Dacron graft between the vaginal wall and urethropelvic ligament, in close proximity to the bladder neck. The Gittes type of needle suspension includes the whole vaginal wall (including epithelium) and the urethropelvic ligaments. The Raz suspension enters the retropubic space, and permanent sutures include the vaginal wall without the epithelium and the pubocervical and medial edges of the urethropelvic ligaments.

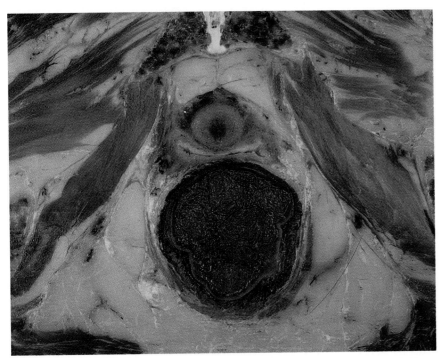

FIGURE 1–19. The intrinsic urethral structure and anatomic support as seen in a fresh-frozen cadaver section. The urethra is anchored to the lateral pelvic wall by a fibrous structure (urethropelvic ligament) where the levator muscles insert into the obturator fascia (tendinous arc). The vaginal wall follows the contour of the periurethral fascia and urethropelvic ligaments.

The Intrinsic Urethral Mechanism

Knowledge of urethral anatomy is also of great importance in understanding stress urinary incontinence. The urethra consists largely of a rich vascular sponge surrounded by a coat of smooth muscle and fibroelastic tissue. Built up of loosely woven connective tissue with tiny smooth muscle bundles scattered throughout and an elaborate vascular plexus, the submucosa creates the so-called "washer effect" for the continence mechanism (Figs. 1–19 and 1–20). Functionally, the surrounding smooth muscle coat maintains this mechanism by directing submucosal expansile pressures inward toward the mucosa. This highly efficient mucosal seal, we believe, is a major contributor to the closure mechanism of the urethra and thus an important aspect of the normal urinary continence mechanism. The plasticity of this structure normally allows perfect continence even when a grooved sound is inserted into the urethra. This "mucosal sphincter" is under hormonal control, and lack of estrogen at menopause leads to atrophy and substitution of the vascular supply by fibrous tissue. Multiple operations, trauma, radiation, and neurogenic disease also can affect the ability to achieve a perfect seal. When this mechanism is lost, stress incontinence results. Simple bladder neck and proximal urethral suspension in these cases will not achieve continence; treatment must be aimed at providing coaptation and urethral compression and not just restoring anatomic support.

An effective means of evaluating this aspect of continence is not readily available. Urethral pressure profilometry, although commonly used, has been found to be nonspecific, poorly reproducible, and fraught with artifacts. Measurement of Valsalva leak pressure is a useful tool with which to assess urethral resistance.

FIGURE 1–20. Transection of the proximal urethra clearly shows its histologic structure—an inner infolded mucosal layer and a rich, spongy vascular cushion surrounded by a thin fibromuscular layer.

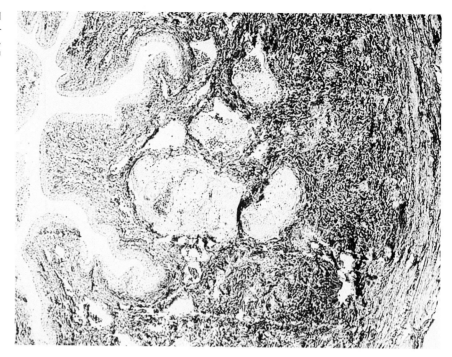

POSTERIOR VAGINAL SUPPORT

A complex fascial and muscular arrangement provides support to the vagina, rectum, perineum, and anal sphincter. Whereas the fascial support includes the prerectal and pararectal fasciae, there are two levels of muscular support: (1) the pelvic floor (levator sling—in particular its pubococcygeal portion), and (2) the urogenital diaphragm, including the bulbocavernosus muscle, the superficial and deep transverse perineal muscles, the external anal sphincter, and the central tendon of the perineum.

In the normally supported patient in the erect position, two vaginal angles of support can be described (Fig. 1–21). In its midportion, the vagina forms a posterior angle of approximately 110 degrees. This angulation indicates the point where the vagina crosses the pelvic floor. The proximal half of the vagina is practically in a horizontal plane resting over the rectum and the levator plate. The second angle defines the relationship between the distal half of the vagina and the vertical line. This angle is approximately 45 degrees, reflecting again the degree of support of the levator muscles and urogenital diaphragm.

In patients with pelvic floor relaxation (Fig. 1–22), the normal anatomic support is lost. The levator plate relaxes (convex instead of horizontal), the levator hiatus enlarges (Fig. 1–23), and the normal midvaginal angulation of 110 degrees disappears. The distal half of the vagina is no longer 45 degrees from the vertical. The vagina is now rotated downward and posteriorly and is no longer in a high supported horizontal position; herniation of the rectum may ensue.

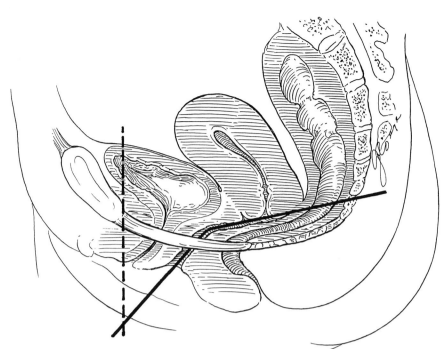

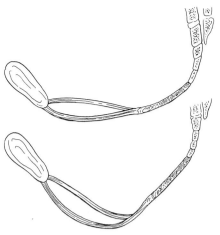

FIGURE 1–21. Lateral view of the vaginal support. The proximal half of the vagina rests almost horizontally over the levator plate, forming a posterior angle of approximately 110 degrees with the distal half of the vagina. The distal half of the vaginal canal has an angle of inclination of approximately 45 degrees with the vertical axis. (From Walsh PC, Gittes RF, Perlmutter AD, Stamey TA: Campbell's Urology, 6th ed. Philadelphia, WB Saunders, 1992.)

FIGURE 1–22. *Top*, The normal supported, almost horizontal, pelvic floor and levator hiatus. The vaginal canal, the urethra, and the rectum cross over this hiatus. Together with the respective fasciae, the levator muscle contributes to the support of the pelvic organs. *Bottom*, In patients with pelvic floor relaxation, the hiatus is wider and the levator plate is relaxed and weakened. In patients with stress urinary incontinence and pelvic floor relaxation, repair or support of the anterior vaginal wall without repair of the levator plate may cause the other pelvic organs to prolapse further (rectocele, enterocele, or uterine prolapse). (From Walsh PC, Gittes RF, Perlmutter AD, Stamey TA: Campbell's Urology, 6th ed. Philadelphia, WB Saunders, 1992.)

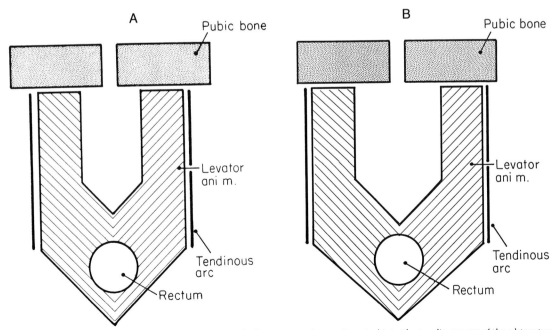

FIGURE 1–23. Diagram of the pelvic floor. In A, the levator muscles are inserted into the tendinous arc of the obturator muscles. They fuse medially behind and just before the rectum and then separate to form a hiatus through which the vagina and uretha cross. B, In patients with pelvic floor relaxation, the hiatus is wider, the medial margin of the levators is separated, and the prerectal support is lax. (From Walsh PC, Gittes RF, Perlmutter AD, Stamey TA: Campbell's Urology, 6th ed. Philadelphia, WB Saunders, 1992.)

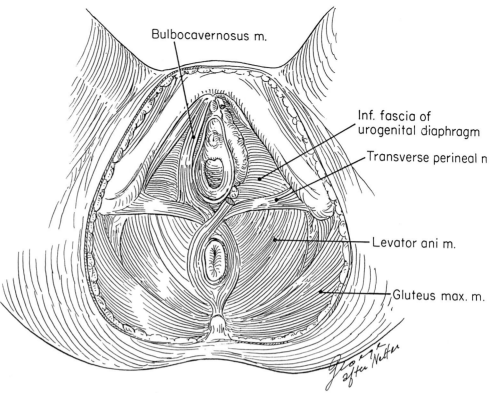

Bulbocavernosus m.

Inf. fascia of urogenital diaphragm

Transverse perineal n

Levator ani m.

Gluteus max. m.

FIGURE 1–24. The perineum is divided in anterior and posterior portions, with the dividing line being the transverse perineal muscle. The musculature of the posterior perineum consists of the external anal sphincter and the levator muscle. The anterior perineum has two levels. The deeper anterior perineum consists mainly of the levator plate, whereas the superficial perineum includes the muscles of the urogenital diaphragm: the bulbocavernous, superficial, and deep transverse perineum and the central tendon of the perineum. (From Walsh PC, Gittes RF, Perlmutter AD, Stamey TA: Campbell's Urology, 6th ed. Philadelphia, WB Saunders, 1992.)

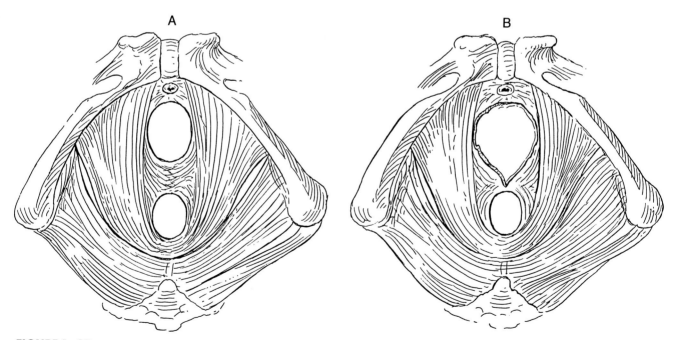

FIGURE 1–25. Perineal view of the levator plate without the muscles of the urogenital diaphragm. In A, the levator hiatus is relatively narrow, allowing passage of the vagina, urethra, and rectum. Fibers of the levator are crossing in the midline before the rectum, providing support. B, In patients with pelvic floor relaxation, the levator hiatus is wider, and the crossing prerectal fibers are attenuated and laterally retracted. (From Walsh PC, Gittes RF, Perlmutter AD, Stamey TA: Campbell's Urology, 6th ed. Philadelphia, WB Saunders, 1992.)

In patients with damage to the second level of muscular support (the perineal or urogenital diaphragm, (Fig. 1–24), the vaginal outlet is wider, and the distance between the urethra and posterior fourchette is increased. Different degrees of perineal tear may be seen: from minimal with only a small separation of the perineum to a severe degree in which the perineal structures have disappeared and the vaginal wall reaches the anterior rectal wall.

Corrective surgery of the posterior vaginal wall should include (1) correction of the rectocele by reinforcement of the attenuated prerectal and pararectal fasciae, (2) repair of the defect of the levator muscles by narrowing the size of the levator hiatus and providing a horizontal supporting plate for the proximal half of the vagina, and (3) repair of the urogenital diaphragm (musculature of the perineum) providing normal introital size and improved vaginal support (Figs. 1–25 and 1–26).

Support of both anterior and posterior vaginal walls must be corrected at the time of stress incontinence operation. Repair of anterior vaginal wall prolapse (bladder neck suspension or cystocele repair) without simultaneous repair of posterior vaginal wall defect (levator plate) may lead to significant anatomic changes. The anterior vaginal wall displacement to a high supported position will transfer the vaginal dome and posterior wall to a most dependent position in the pelvis, and changes in abdominal pressure will tend to exaggerate a prior rectocele, enterocele, or uterine prolapse.

Repair of pelvic floor relaxation also may be important in the outcome of stress incontinence surgery. Transmission of intra-abdominal forces to the urethra is an important mechanism compensating for sudden changes in abdominal pressure. A strong pelvic floor supports the pelvic organs for efficient transmission of this pressure. Pelvic floor repair will result in better continence for the patient.

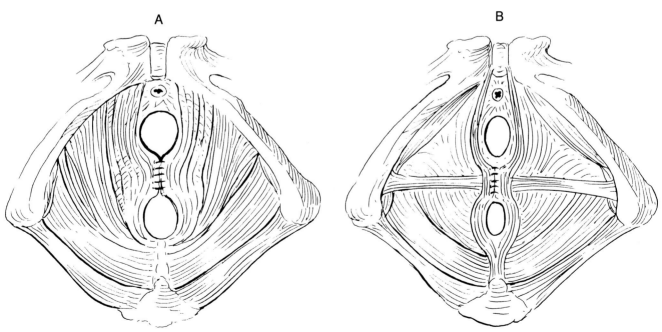

A   B

FIGURE 1–26. The goal of surgery in posterior repair is A, to reconstruct the levator plate by approximation of its prerectal fibers, and B, to repair the urogenital diaphragm by approximation of the bulbocavernous and transverse muscles, external anal sphincter, and central tendon of the perineum to a normal anatomic position. (From Walsh PC, Gittes RF, Perlmutter AD, Stamey TA: Campbell's Urology, 6th ed. Philadelphia, WB Saunders, 1992.)

Uterine Support

A good description of vaginal dome and uterine support can be found in a standard textbook of anatomy. The most important supporting structures of the uterus are the sacrouterine, broad, and cardinal ligaments. The sacrouterine ligaments are posteriorly located and run from the cervix to the side of the sacrum. At the level of the cervix, they fuse with the posterior aspect of the cardinal ligaments. The broad ligaments are superiorly located and covered by anterior and posterior folds of peritoneum attaching the lateral walls of the uterine body to the lateral pelvic wall. The broad ligament contains the fallopian tubes, round and ovarian ligaments, uterine arteries, and ovarian vessels. The cardinal ligaments were described earlier. They are the most important uterine supporting structure. Relaxation of the cardinal ligaments facilitates the formation of cystocele, enterocele, and vaginal vault prolapse.

Summary

Our findings help us divide true stress urinary incontinence into (1) that due to anatomic malposition of an intact sphincteric unit, and (2) that secondary to insufficiency of the urethral closing mechanism or intrinsic urethral damage. The goal of surgery for anatomic incontinence is to elevate and support the bladder neck in a high, fixed retropubic position by resuspension of the urethropelvic ligaments, whereas the goal of surgery in patients with intrinsic damage is to provide coaptation and compression of the urethra in order to restore its sealing function.

Repair of pelvic floor relaxation seems to be important in the outcome of stress incontinence surgery. It provides a strong base plate, the pelvic floor, in which intra-abdominal pressures are more efficiently transmitted to the proximal urethral mechanism. It also restores the vaginal axis to normal, protecting the vaginal dome and posterior vaginal wall from prolapsing.

INSTRUMENTATION

FOR VAGINAL

SURGERY

Successful vaginal surgery requires proper instrumentation. This chapter reviews some of the instruments that we have found most useful.

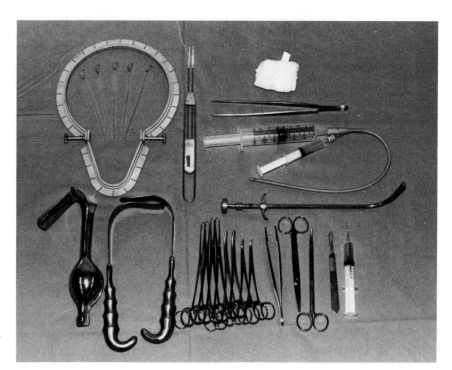

FIGURE 2–1. In addition to the basic tray for vaginal surgery, we include a weighted speculum, right-angle retractors, Allis and hemostatic clamps, Bonney and long Russian forceps, syringe with normal saline for injection, Lowsley retractor for suprapubic cystostomy, Raz double-pronged needle for suspension, Scott ring retractor, and vaginal packing. A few special instruments and suture material will be described further in detail.

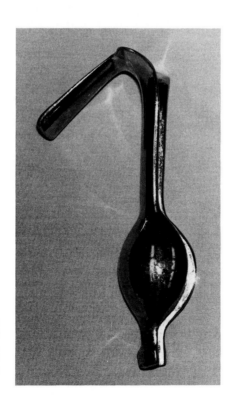

FIGURE 2–2. A weighted vaginal speculum (Auvard) with a 45-degree angle is the most commonly used. In high vesicovaginal fistula, a longer speculum may be needed. A glove should be inserted at the end of the speculum to collect blood.

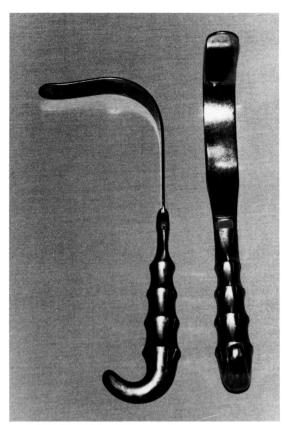

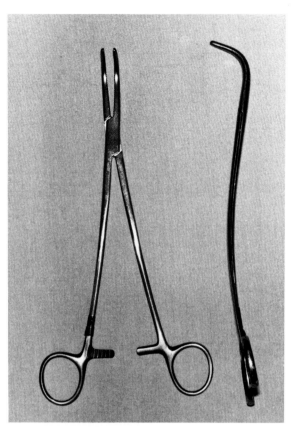

FIGURE 2–3. A right-angle retractor (Heaney) is used for proper exposure of the vaginal vault. It is also useful in cases of narrow introitus or short vagina when the weighted speculum cannot be used. A weight can be attached to its hooked end to facilitate the exposure.

FIGURE 2–4. Right-angle clamp used for vaginal hysterectomy. Its long tip allows for easy isolation of the sacrouterine and cardinal ligaments and the uterine pedicle.

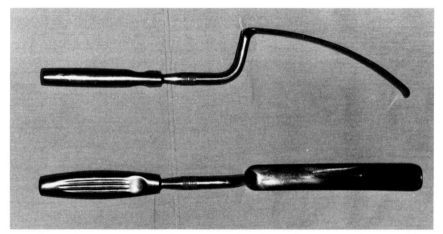

FIGURE 2–5. The Breisky-Navratil retractor used for deep exposure as in sacrospinalis fixation of the vaginal vault. Its shape allows for medial retraction of the rectum without interfering with application of the supporting sutures in the sacrospinous ligament.

FIGURE 2–6. Raz double-pronged needle used for bladder neck suspension. The distance between the points is 1 cm. The tip of the needle is transferred under finger control and is stopped by the anterior abdominal wall fascia. The inner segment of the ligature carrier can be slid over the external support, extending the tip of the needle, under finger control, toward the vaginal area.

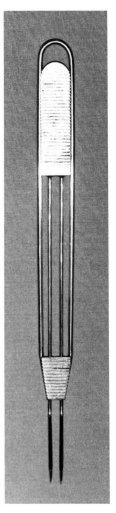

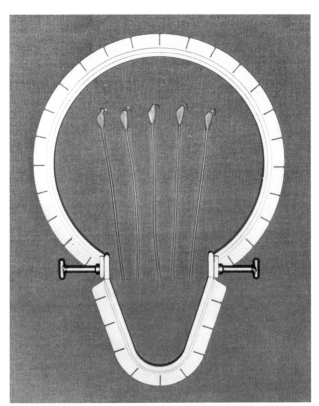

FIGURE 2–7. The Scott ring retractor with hooks is extremely useful in vaginal surgery. Except for a simple bladder neck suspension, it is used for most vaginal procedures, such as rectocele, enterocele and perineal repair; vaginal hysterectomy; grade IV cystocele repair; repair of vesicovaginal fistula; and so on.

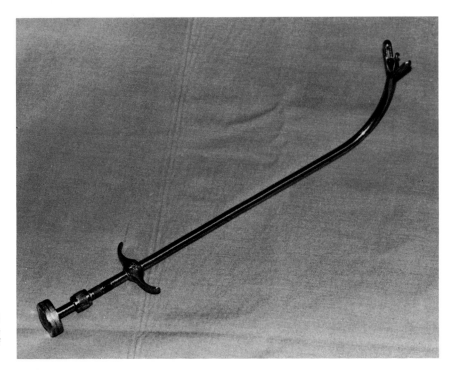

FIGURE 2–8. Curved Lowsley retractor used for insertion of a Foley suprapubic catheter. The tip of a Foley catheter is grasped by the jaws of the retractor and transferred to the bladder.

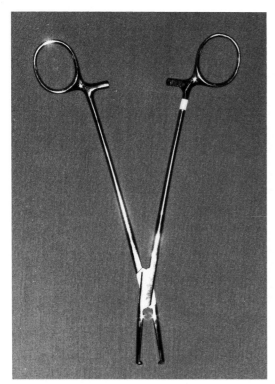

FIGURE 2–9. Curved Phaneuf clamp, used to clamp and ligate the cardinal, sacrouterine, and broad ligaments during hysterectomy. The teeth at the tips do not allow undesired escape of tissue during hemostasis.

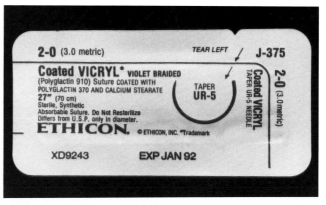

FIGURE 2–10. Coated Vicryl suture 2-0 (Ethicon) on a tapered UR-5 needle. The shape of the needle allows better placement of sutures high in the vagina, especially in the repair of vesicovaginal fistula.

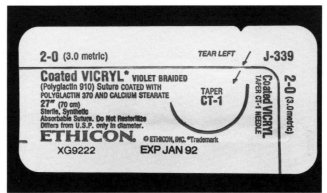

FIGURE 2–11. Coated Vicryl suture 2-0 (Ethicon) on a tapered CT-I needle. This suture is used for closure of the vaginal wall, rectocele, and perineal repair.

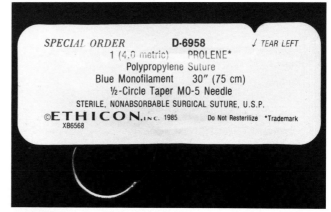

FIGURE 2–12. Number I polypropylene monofilament nonabsorbable suture (Prolene, Ethicon) on a half-circle, tapered MO-5 needle. This suture is used for bladder neck and bladder suspension operations. The shape and strength of the needle make it useful in repeat operations when the patient has extensive scarring. This needle size is the most appropriate for most patients. Number I monofilament polybutester (Novafil, Davis and Geck) in a T-40 or T-56 needle also can be used.

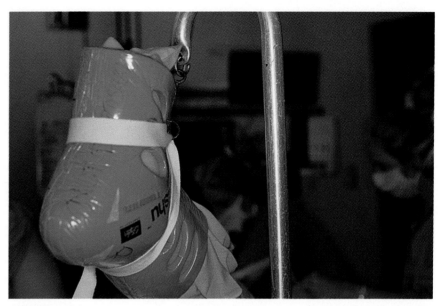

FIGURE 2–13. Ankle stirrups are placed perpendicular to the table so that no contact of the lower extremity with the vertical bar can occur. The special boots are used to support and protect the feet and ankles, preventing undesired pressure or accidental drop of the feet from the stirrups.

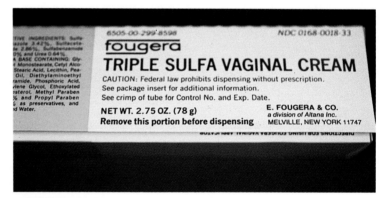

FIGURE 2–14. Triple-sulfa vaginal cream used for soaking the vaginal pack after every routine vaginal operation.

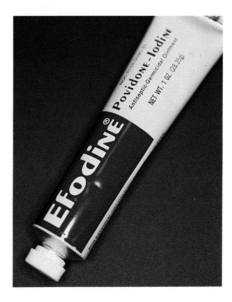

FIGURE   2–15. Povidone-iodine   cream used for soaking the vaginal pack.

Operating Room Card

Bladder Neck Suspension and Cystocele or Rectocele Repair

Surgeon: SR   *Gloves:* 7 pr.   *Skin Prep:* Iodophor/Vaginal

Position: Lithotomy with candy-cane stirrups, foam boots to feet

Drapes: Vaginal-perineal peripack

Sutures and Needles:

2-0 silk on #4 Mayo trocar to sew the drapes
  (5 needed)
2-0 Vicryl CT-1 for vaginal closure
4-0 Vicryl F-82 for skin
2-0 nylon FSLX for suprapubic catheter
No. 1 Prolene D-6958 Ethicon (special order)

Instruments and Equipment:

Basic minor
Bonney forceps
Curved Lowsley traction clamp
Long Allis clamps
Long Russian forceps
Auvard weighted speculum
Heaney retractors
Cystoscope and cysto tubing
Double-pronged ligature carrier
Vaginal pack with triple sulfa cream or Betadine
Peripad and belt
2 Foley catheters, French 16
2 urine bags for suprapubic and urethral catheters
Scott ring retractor with 6 hooks (for rectocele or
  cystocele)

Dressing:

4 × 8 gauze squares and Micropore tape
Vaginal packing
Peripad and belt

Vaginal Hysterectomy Add-on

2 angled Phaneuf clamps
2 Gray cystic right-angle clamps
Lahey tenaculum
Single-pronged tenaculum
Long Allis clamps

Sacrospinalis Fixation Add-on

Breisky-Navratil retractor
No. 1 Vicryl on CT-2 needle

Closure of Vesicovaginal Fistula

Long Metzenbaum scissors
Male urethral sound for dilation of the tract
8–10 French Foley catheter
Diluted indigo carmine solution

3

SUPRAPUBIC CYSTOSTOMY; PLACEMENT OF A FOLEY CATHETER USING THE LOWSLEY RETRACTOR

INDICATIONS

Temporary or permanent bypass of the urethra via suprapubic catheter drainage of the bladder is an important adjunct in many pelvic operations. The procedure described here is simple and allows for accurate and safe placement of a Foley catheter of any type and size. Suprapubic catheterization using a Lowsley retractor (Fig. 3–1) is more convenient for the patient, reducing hospital stay and cost.

The other catheters available for suprapubic cystostomy tend to leak from the site of bladder puncture and thus cannot be plugged in the immediate postoperative period. Using a Foley catheter enables one to pull the intravesical balloon against the abdominal wall, preventing leakage. The catheter can be plugged 12 to 24 hours after surgery, and the patient can be discharged without the inconvenience of a bag.

CONTRAINDICATIONS

Cystostomy should not be performed on patients with an active infection of the lower abdominal wall. Prior bowel disease or cystoplasty increases the risk of bowel perforation, and cystostomy should be performed only with extreme caution.

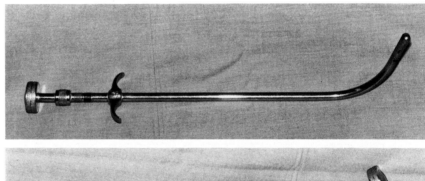

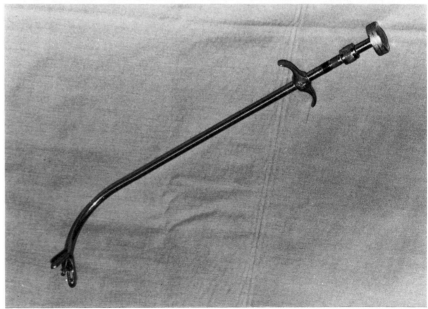

FIGURE 3–1. The Lowsley retractor. The jaws are opened by rotating the knob at the instrument's base.

SURGICAL TECHNIQUE

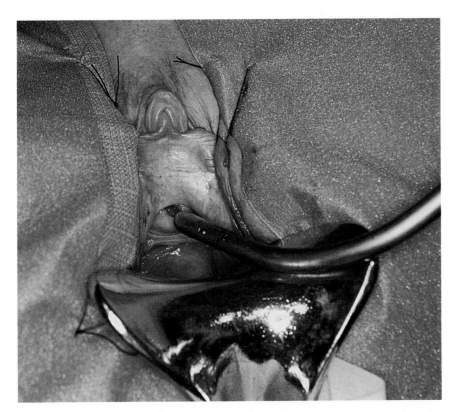

STEP 1

The patient is positioned in the lithotomy position and the closed Lowsley retractor is passed into the bladder through the urethra. The bladder wall is tented toward the anterior abdominal wall by forward pressure on the retractor, which is held firmly to avoid posterior pressure or angulation of the urethra.

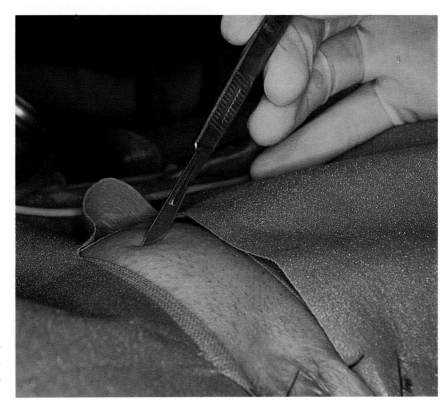

STEP 2

A suprapubic stab incision is made over the tip of the retractor through the anterior abdominal wall, including the rectus fascia.

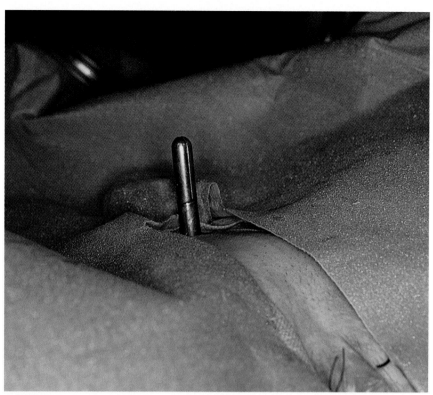

STEP 3

The tip of the Lowsley retractor is transferred through the abdominal wall incision.

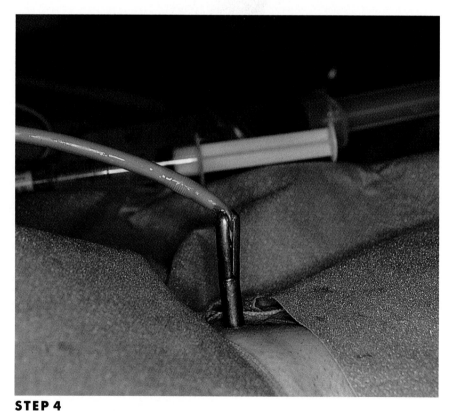

STEP 4

A catheter of any size (in general we use 16 French Foley catheters) is grasped with the tip of the Lowsley retractor and secured between the prongs.

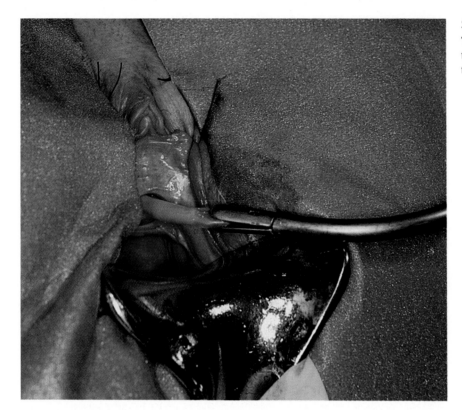

STEP 5
The retractor and catheter are pulled back through the bladder and should exit through the urethral meatus.

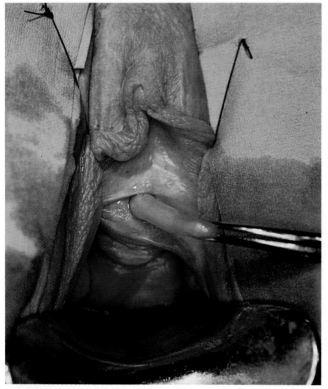

STEP 6
The Lowsley retractor is removed. With its tip anchored to a hemostat clamp, the catheter is pulled back into the bladder.

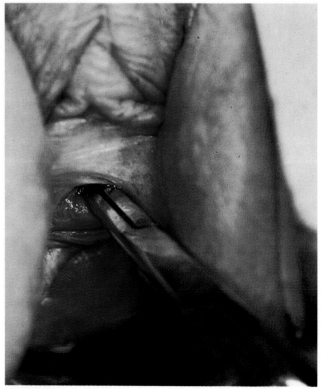

STEP 7
After proper positioning of the catheter tip in the bladder, the balloon of the Foley catheter is inflated and irrigated to confirm its position within the bladder. Only then is the clamp removed.

Mild traction is applied to the catheter, and a wet gauze square is tied around it, against the stab wound. This maneuver will tamponade any bleeding from the bladder or in the perivesical space. At the end of the operative procedure, the wet gauze is removed, and the catheter is fixed in place with number 2-0 nylon suture.

INTRAOPERATIVE COMPLICATIONS

Potential complications with percutaneous suprapubic cystostomy catheters include placement of the catheter outside the bladder or within the urethra, excessive bleeding in the perivesical space, and injury to intra-abdominal viscera. Injury to intra-abdominal viscera is avoided by the approximation of the bladder wall to the anterior abdominal wall during the insertion process.

A particular risk of this procedure is the possible damage to the urethra if excessive angulation or posterior pressure is applied to the urethra with the Lowsley retractor. This risk is avoided by forward pressure on the retractor.

POSTOPERATIVE CARE

Beyond the routine for suprapubic catheterization, no special postoperative care is necessary. The catheter may be used to empty the bladder, to measure postvoid residual urine, and to irrigate blood clots or mucous threads if necessary.

POSTOPERATIVE COMPLICATIONS

Postoperative bleeding can be avoided by gentle traction on the catheter. A faulty catheter may dislodge in the postoperative period, requiring transurethral drainage.

COMPLICATIONS OF VAGINAL SURGERY

The best way to manage surgical complications is to prevent them. Prevention requires exact knowledge of a patient's history, knowledge of human topographic anatomy, and thorough awareness of the difficulties that may arise during the planned operation. Being prepared enables accurate recognization of a complication. Whether or not the surgeon has precise knowledge of all anatomic details and great surgical skill, unanticipated problems may still occur.

Preoperative diagnostic studies, like a voiding cystogram, intravenous urogram, or ultrasonography, enable the urinary tract to be visualized prior to transvaginal surgery; interpretation of the findings may ensure that potential intraoperative problems are foreseen.

Timely recognition of a complication can prevent unfortunate late sequelae. Satisfactory results are much more likely if the injury is recognized and repaired at the time of occurrence and not at a later date.

The reported incidence of injury of the urinary or intestinal tract during gynecologic surgery is 5 to 8 per cent.

Surgical complications can be separated into those that are intraoperative, those that are early (complications not recognized at the time of surgery), and late complications. We will discuss each of the complications separately as they apply to the ureter, bladder, vagina, and bowel.

Ureteric Injuries

Intraoperative ureteric injury during vaginal surgery occurs rarely, considering the total number of vaginal procedures performed. It is suggested that this incidence is less than 0.5 per cent, although precise numbers are not known. Risk factors for ureteric injury include prior abdominal operation, vaginal prolapse such as enterocele or large cystocele, and multiple prior vaginal operations. The importance of careful cystoscopic examination of the ureteric orifices after injection of indigo carmine in any vaginal surgery close to the ureter must be emphasized. If the dye is not visualized, retrograde catheterization, retrograde pyelogram, or ureteroscopy should be performed.

Ureteric injury has many causes, such as clamping, stitching, ligatures, incision, coagulation, and total severance.

Short-term clamping of the ureter does not lead to ischemic damage. In general, the clamping is incomplete and some periureteric tissue is also captured. If hard clamps have been used and the ureter clamped for a short period of time, a double J stent should be inserted and remain in place for a period of at least 1 week after surgery. If the ureter is cross clamped for a longer period (more than 1 hour), it must be assumed that more extensive damage has occurred. A lesion of this nature requires exposure of this part of the ureter and resection of the damaged area.

A small ureterotomy may be easily corrected if the cut edges can be seen clearly. To preserve the blood supply, care must be taken that periureteric tissue is not dissected too extensively. Interrupted fine 4-0 or 5-0 absorbable sutures should be used. The ureter should be intubated and the repair properly drained. This drain should exit from the suprapubic area and not the vagina.

If the ureter has been captured incompletely by a suture that is removed immediately, surgical repair is not required. Nevertheless, a double J stent should be inserted, because we can never know for sure the extent of the ischemic damage. Upon removal of the injuring suture, the ureter should be observed to estimate its color and shape. If the affected area is discolored, narrow, and adynamic, a resection of the ischemic area is recommended.

Reanastomosis of severed ends of a ureter may be performed using an oblique or spatulated technique. A normal thin, nondilated ureter can be easily reanastomosed with five or six interrupted absorbable 4-0 or 5-0 sutures. Too many sutures or very tight tying may lead to ischemia of the anastomotic site. The anastomosis should be properly drained and a stent inserted for proper modeling. With proper exposure, the end-to-end anatomosis or ureteric reimplantation may be done transvaginally, but as a rule it is simpler and safer to perform the repair transabdominally. Proper dissection of the proximal ureter will provide a tension-free line of suture. If the ureteral length is adequate, a direct antireflux ureteroneocystostomy may be performed. If the proximal ureter is too short, a psoas hitch or Boari-type bladder flap can be used for the antireflux reimplantation.

In the postoperative period, the main manifestation of an unrecognized ureteric injury is obstruction or extravasation. Postoperative flank pain and tenderness of the costovertebral angle are signs of ureteric obstruction. Very often postoperative analgesia may mask these symptoms. In this case a rise in the creatinine level, diffuse abdominal pain, or paralytic ileus after vaginal surgery can be the main presentation. Urinary extravasation may explain the lack of pain in cases of complete ureteric obstruction or injury. Renal ultrasound may discover hydronephrosis or a perirenal or pelvic urinary collection. Intravenous pyelogram may reveal poor kidney visualization, hydronephrosis, or a nonfunctional kidney. In cases of complete or partial ureteric injury, the pyelogram may be normal, and contrast material can be seen outside the urinary tract in the late films.

When the diagnosis of ureteral obstruction is made, in particular if it is incomplete, an attempt to pass a stent should be the first choice. If the defect cannot be passed with the stent, it may be possible to overcome the obstruction with use of the ureteroscope. Under direct vision a guide wire may be inserted and a stent advanced in place. If the diagnosis of complete ureteric obstruction is made, two approaches are possible: primary repair or temporary percutaneous nephrostomy with secondary operation at a later time. A temporary nephrostomy may in rare cases avoid a secondary operation by allowing the sutures around the ureter to be reabsorbed, spontaneously resolving the obstruction.

Bladder Injury

The cause of intraoperative bladder injury may be excision, incision, excessive coagulation, or clamping of the bladder wall. Risk factors include multiple operations in the past, tissue atrophy, and radiation. Most of the lesions occur at the bladder base but, with the increased use of needle bladder neck suspension, lesions of the bladder neck have become common. Prevention of bladder injury includes delicate dissection, use of the known anatomic landmarks, and avoidance of undue retraction or fulguration.

A plugged transurethral and/or suprapubic catheter at the time of surgery is recommended. The urethral catheter aids location of the urethra and trigone. During surgery urine collects in the bladder, so the appearance of bloody urine that was clear at the beginning of the operation should make the surgeon suspect bladder injury. Urine will appear in the surgical field if the bladder lumen has been opened inadvertently. Normal saline, methylene blue or indigo carmine solutions may be instilled to locate the site of the lesion.

If the injury is diagnosed at the time of operation, the bladder wall must be exposed sufficiently. A two-layer closure is required, with a running inner layer and an interrupted second layer of perivesical fascia. If required, a fibrofatty labial flap can be used to reinforce the repair. On completion of the closure, cystoscopy must ensure that the ureters are patent, and bladder irrigation must be performed to demonstrate the watertightness of the suture lines. A drain to the area of injury is recommended. It may be inserted by passing a long clamp from the suprapubic to the vaginal area under finger control. The end of the clamp grasps the end of the Penrose drain, transferring it to the suprapubic area. After proper positioning of the drain, the vaginal wall may be closed. Uninterrupted suprapubic sutures and urethral drainage of urine for at least 10 days are very important to avoid fistula formation. A cystogram should confirm good bladder emptying and the absence of extravasation.

With the increased use of needle suspensions, penetration of the bladder by nonabsorbable sutures is common. It is extremely important to make a careful cystoscopic examination of the bladder at the end of the operation. The sutures can be easily removed and repositioned without complications. On rare occasions, delayed perforation of the bladder may occur weeks or months after the operation. The symptoms of severe urgency and frequency and urinary infections, together with cystoscopy, confirm the presence of a foreign body in the bladder (see Figs. 4–2, 4–3). Long-term sutures in the bladder can present as stones fixed to the bladder wall. In general, the sutures can be removed under local anesthesia in the surgeon's office, using cystoscopic scissors.

Bladder injury unrecognized at the time of surgery is one of the most important complications of vaginal surgery. Prolonged hematuria, leakage of urine despite bladder drainage, or severe pain in the bladder area may indicate bladder injury. A cystogram may confirm extravasation of urine, and cystoscopy will confirm the location and extent of the bladder injury. Adequate bladder drainage should be obtained and on rare occasions percutaneous insertion of a drain may be required. Because of the extent of the bladder injury, some patients will develop a vesicovaginal fistula in spite of proper drainage. After an adequate period of conservative therapy, the fistula may be approached surgically.

Bowel Injury

Bowel injury at the time of vaginal surgery is another major complication of vaginal surgery, particularly if the patient had no bowel preparation prior to operation. Repair of iatrogenic injury of the colon or small bowel follows established criteria of general surgery. If the patient had a proper bowel preparation and the injury is easily identified, a primary repair can be performed. A multiple-layer closure should be done, and dilatation of the anal sphincter is recommended.

Extensive damage of the rectum with spilling of stool matter into the surgical field requires a protective colostomy together with the repair. Proper use of vaginal retractors and delicate dissection over the rectal area can prevent rectal injury. Risk factors for rectal damage include multiple prior operations, radiation, and bowel disease. Whenever a rectocele or enterocele repair is contemplated, the lower bowel must be properly prepared. We routinely insert per rectum a gauze square soaked in Betadine solution. This packing permits palpation of the rectal wall at the time of vaginal repair, facilitates the dissection, and may help prevent rectal injury.

Nerve Injury

Denervation of the bladder can occur after extensive vaginal surgery, which may contribute to postoperative urinary retention. The etiology of bladder instability after vaginal surgery is not clear and is not related to bladder wall denervation.

Because of the proximity of the pudendal nerve to the sacrospinalis ligament, injury can occur during sacrospinalis fixation for vaginal vault prolapse. Proper exposure of the paravaginal space and palpation of the ischial spine may avoid this complication. The fixation sutures must be placed at least 2 cm medial to the ischial spine.

Peroneal nerve palsy or femoral neuropathy is rare after vaginal surgery. The patient should be carefully positioned to avoid nerve injury, but the lithotomy position itself may create nerve injury in spite of proper support. Recovery from this injury is usually spontaneous but will sometimes be prolonged over several months.

Bleeding

The prevention of intraoperative or postoperative bleeding begins prior to operation. A prior history of unusual response to trauma or previous operation must be sought. Medications such as aspirin or other nonsteroidal anti-inflammatory drugs should be stopped at least 2 weeks prior to surgery. The platelet count, prothrombin time, and partial thromboplastin time give a good estimate of clotting abnormalities. Bleeding time may be determined as well.

Ignoring intraoperative bleeding with the hope that venous bleeding can be stopped by extrinsic pressure is dangerous. The retropubic and perirectal spaces are not confined and they will not tamponade a venous bleeding. At the end of the operation, and prior to closure of the vaginal wall, the surgical field must be clear. Coagulation should be used with extreme caution for defined bleeders; suture ligatures are preferred. Minor vaginal oozing can be controlled by the use of a vaginal packing. If bleeding is more profuse, a Foley catheter with a 50- to 60-ml balloon can be inserted against the packing (Fig. 4–1).

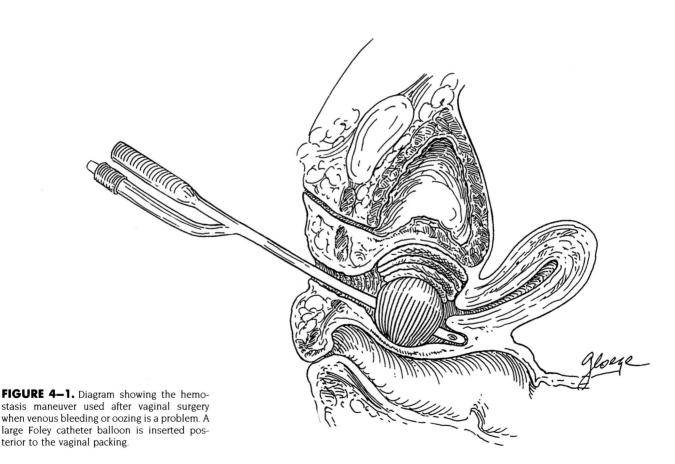

FIGURE 4–1. Diagram showing the hemostasis maneuver used after vaginal surgery when venous bleeding or oozing is a problem. A large Foley catheter balloon is inserted posterior to the vaginal packing.

A low blood pressure, tachycardia, and a drop in the hematocrit count without external vaginal bleeding are clear signs of retropubic or retroperitoneal bleeding. Resuscitation maneuvers are used, and re-exploration and even a laparotomy may be required. Ultrasound or computed tomography scan may help in location of the bleeding area. In special cases pelvic angiography and embolization of an arterial bleeder may correct the problem.

A late onset of bleeding, 5 or more days after vaginal operation, is rare. It will respond usually by applying a vaginal packing. The bleeding may result from local infection, requiring antibiotic therapy.

Thromboembolic Complications

The operative risk of deep vein thrombosis and pulmonary emboli after vaginal surgery is not high when compared with thoracic or abdominal intervention. Still it is a known complication and must be prevented.

The positioning of the patient on the operating table must be watched carefully. Compression of the lower extremities by the supporting stirrups can generate stasis and a tendency to venous thrombosis. We strongly recommend the use of ankle stirrups to avoid this problem. The use of elastic or hydraulic stockings may improve circulation, particularly in the postoperative period. The patient should be encouraged to move her legs freely while in bed, and early mobilization is encouraged—if possible the morning or the day after the operation. Excessive analgesia and sedation may impair mobility and increase the tendency for stasis.

High-risk patients with a prior history of venous thrombosis or emboli should receive anticoagulation therapy in the perioperative period. A low dose of 5000 units of subcutaneous heparin, two or three times a day, is very effective and can be easily reversed if required. If thrombosis or emboli are clinically evident, intravenous heparinization should be used. After a loading dose, continuous heparin is given intravenously, starting with 1000 units an hour, with careful control of the partial thromboplastin time.

Infection

The vagina is potentially contaminated by various types of bacteria. The flora vary with the patient's age, time of her cycle, sexual activity, and social environment. Preoperative cleansing of the vagina by douche with antibacterial soaps is recommended to reduce the number of bacteria. Patients with vaginitis, cervicitis, or urinary or urethral infections should be aggressively treated before surgery.

Short-term antibacterial prophylaxis is very effective in vaginal surgery. The first dose is given before the operation and then for a period of 24 to 48 hours afterward. Depending on the antibiotic's half-life, various regimens are equally effective. We use a combination of synthetic penicillins or cephalosporins with an aminoglycoside. This combination has proven antibacterial activity against gram-positive and gram-negative bacteria. Metronidazole is effective against anaerobic organisms and should be used with bowel reconstructive surgery.

Antibacterial medication in the presence of indwelling catheters has a potential to select resistant organisms, accelerating the growth of highly resistant nosocomial bacteria. Antibacterial prophylaxis is advocated in the elderly or high-risk patient. If these patients have obesity, diabetes, or cardiac or lung disease, an outbreak of infection could threaten their lives.

Fever in the first 48 hours after vaginal surgery is a major concern. Lung atelectasis or infection of the intravenous lines should be ruled out. Pelvic and renal ultrasound studies should be performed to rule out urinary tract

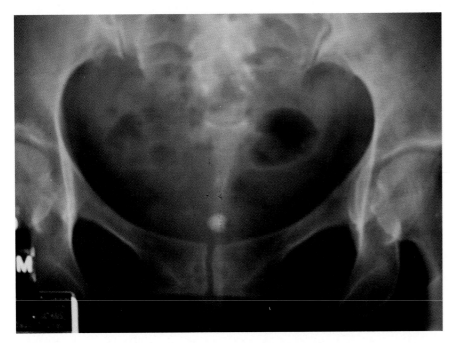

FIGURE 4-2. Radiograph of the pelvis shows a bladder stone in a patient suffering from recurrent urinary tract infections after a Marshall-Marchetti procedure. A nonabsorbable intravesical suture was found to be the nidus for the stone.

obstruction, pelvic collection, or other local pathology. An intravenous pyelogram may reveal ureteric obstruction or fistula. The urine should be cultured for possible urinary tract infection; urinary infection, lumbar pain, and fever are signs of pyelonephritis and should be treated aggressively.

Lower urinary tract infections after surgery are common and respond well to short courses of antibiotics. Recurrent or persistent infection after vaginal surgery requires a detailed evaluation, including cystogram and cystoscopy as indicated.

Prolonged fever after vaginal hysterectomy, sacrospinalis fixation, or rectocele repair can be due to a pelvic abscess. Pelvic ultrasound or computed tomography will confirm the diagnosis. If no response to antibiotics is noted, surgical drainage must be performed.

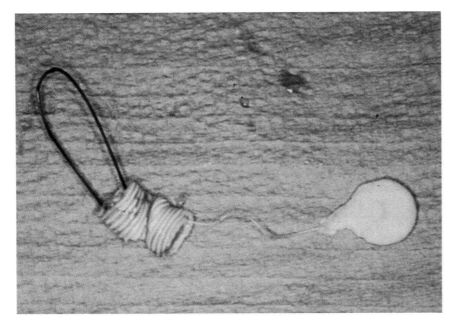

FIGURE 4-3. The Dacron graft and nylon suture have penetrated the bladder (forming a stone), 6 months after a Stamey suspension in a patient suffering from recurrent urinary tract infections.

Vaginal Stenosis or Shortening

Excessive excision of the vaginal wall may lead to narrowing or shortening of the vagina. During rectocele or cystocele repair, the excision of vaginal tissue should be minimal. The excess vaginal wall should be kept in normal saline until the end of the procedure. In case of difficulties in closing the vagina, the vaginal wall can be used as a free graft. Excessive plication or tension of the suture line should be avoided. At the end of a rectocele repair the vaginal wall should be smooth, without bumps or rings, and allow the insertion of at least two fingers with ease. A hematoma of the vaginal wall may lead to late scarring and deformity of the vaginal canal.

Dyspareunia and pelvic pain may indicate vaginal stenosis or shortening, and the physical examination can confirm it. Relaxing longitudinal lateral incisions and horizontal repair are generally sufficient for the correction of mild vaginal stenosis. With large defects or shortening of the vaginal canal, a free skin graft can be used. An expandable intravaginal conformer should be used until the graft is healed.

Urinary Retention

Urinary retention after vaginal surgery is in general a temporary event. Surgical pain, medication, edema, and surgical manipulation of the bladder are all factors in the normal postoperative inability to empty the bladder. Other factors like infection, hematoma, or suspension sutures in close proximity to the bladder neck can induce prolonged urinary retention. Permanent retention is very rare and can result from bladder denervation. Nevertheless a common reason is urethral obstruction (Fig. 4–4). Complete urodynamic evaluation is necessary in this case. This study may reveal a pattern of high pressure and low flow, typical of obstruction. In some instances, the urodynamic examination is negative for obstruction and may reveal the absence of voluntary bladder contractions. If clinically indicated, urethrolysis may be done after several months.

In the postoperative period we prefer the use of a plugged suprapubic catheter, so the patient can attempt to void naturally and check the residue of urine. Intermittent self-catheterization may be painful and difficult in the immediate postoperative period but should be initiated if urinary retention is still present 2 to 3 weeks after operation.

Obstruction after an anterior repair is generally due to extensive and tight plication of the periurethral tissues. After vaginal or abdominal bladder neck suspension, sutures in the proximity of the urethra can impede the normal funneling, relaxation, or shortening of the bladder neck during voiding. A common reason for obstruction after bladder neck suspension is misplacement of the sutures in the midurethral area and not at the bladder neck.

Enterocele and Other Prolapse

Postoperative genital prolapse may recur after properly selected and well-performed vaginal reconstructive surgery. Poor quality of the tissues, vaginal infection or hematoma, and poor general condition may increase the risk for recurrent prolapse.

A secondary enterocele, not present prior to operation, is a complication of any operation that alters the vaginal axis, in particular a bladder neck suspension. Suspension of the anterior vaginal wall will transfer the axis of the vagina, transferring the cul-de-sac to the most dependent part of the pelvis. Changes in intra-abdominal pressure will impact the vaginal vault and facilitate the formation of an enterocele.

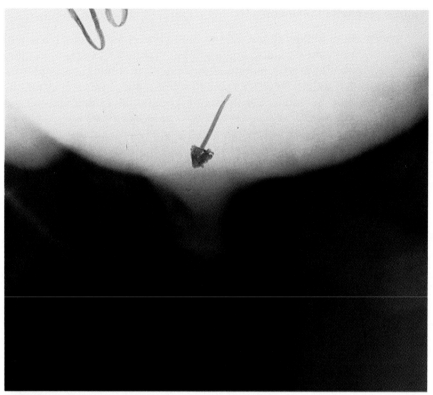

FIGURE 4—4. Voiding cystogram in a patient suffering from severe urinary obstruction after a bladder neck suspension operation. A suture has crossed the area of the proximal urethra. Endoscopic removal of the suture corrected the problem.

Pain

Postoperative pain is a common complication after vaginal surgery. The pain may be suprapubic, vaginal, or rectal.

Suprapubic pain may be related to the insertion of a suprapubic catheter. A cystogram may be required to confirm proper catheter placement and to rule out any complication due to the catheter. Bladder spasms and urgency are often felt as suprapubic pain. Treatment with cholinolytics is required in this case. The most distressing pain in the suprapubic area is the pain related to suspension sutures. The pain is generally transitory and may require much time before it subsides. The cause of this pain may be related to nerve entrapment, sutures tied too tight, or placement of the sutures in a mobile portion of the anterior abdominal wall (movement creates tension over the rectus muscle and fascia). If the suspending sutures are transferred in the midline and placed as close to the pubic bone as possible, suprapubic pain after needle suspension will be very rare.

Vaginal pain after surgery is rare unless hematoma or infection has occurred. An unusual cause of vaginal pain is the inclusion of the levator muscles in a suture line. The patient has pain that increases with intercourse and movement and can be reproduced by vaginal examination of the levator plate. Pain during intercourse may be related to vaginal stenosis or shortening or inflammation of the vaginal wall. A stitch granuloma may lead to chronic sinus infection and pain.

Rectal pain may occur because of hematoma or infection in the rectovaginal space. The diagnosis is evident on physical examination; in rare cases, drainage may be necessary. Extensive perineal repair may lead to temporary perirectal pain.

Bladder Instability

Symptoms of frequency and urgency and urgency incontinence are generally temporary after vaginal surgery. The cause of persistent bladder instability lasting beyond 3 months after operation is not clear (Fig. 4–5). Obstruction may lead to bladder instability in a patient without instability prior to operation, but more often no clear etiology is found. Sling procedures are particularly likely to cause instability symptoms postsurgery. Elderly patients are also at higher risk for bladder instability after a properly selected and well-performed bladder neck suspension. Extensive vaginal operations, particularly large cystocele repair, may cause partial bladder denervation and clear neurologic dysfunction, but this is very rare. Many patients have a mixture of symptoms prior to operation, such as stress and urgency incontinence, and a bladder neck suspension may have controlled only one of the symptoms, stress incontinence, and failed to resolve the instability. Carcinoma in situ should be ruled out in patients with persistent urgency after surgery (Fig. 4–6).

Stress Incontinence

Stress incontinence absent prior to operation may be a complication of vaginal surgery in patients undergoing cystocele repair without concomitant bladder neck suspension. It is recommended that a procedure to elevate the bladder neck and urethra be performed in every case of cystocele and urethral hypermobility (with or without stress incontinence). If this is not done, the urethra will remain hypermobile, facilitating the appearance of stress incontinence.

Recurrent stress incontinence after a transvaginal bladder neck suspension requires a complete evaluation. A common cause is recurrent hypermobility and malposition of the bladder neck and urethra (Fig. 4–7). In this case, the simple repositioning of the sphincteric unit to a high normally supported position will cure the incontinence. In other instances the recurrent incontinence occurs with a well-supported urethra and bladder neck. In this case the cause of recurrent stress incontinence is not anatomic malposition but rather intrinsic sphincter dysfunction of a normally supported urethra. Procedures like bulking injections or sling procedures are used for this condition (see Chapter 5, Section D, on sling procedures).

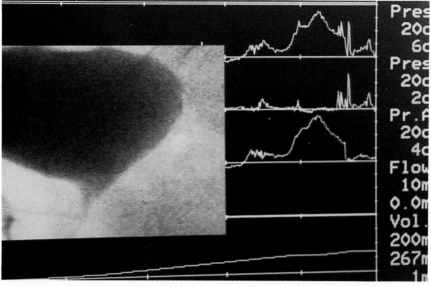 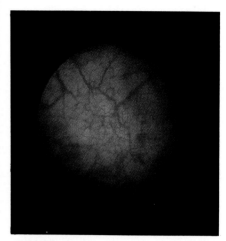

FIGURE 4—5. Video urodynamic evaluation of a patient suffering from severe incontinence after a stress incontinence operation. The upper graph records bladder pressure; just below it the abdominal pressures and the true detrusor pressures are obtained by electronic substraction. Flow was not recorded. The patient had severe, early filling bladder instability, requiring medication.

FIGURE 4—6. Cystoscopy findings of a patient suffering from persistent frequency and urgency after a successful bladder neck suspension operation. Biopsy of the lesions revealed carcinoma in situ.

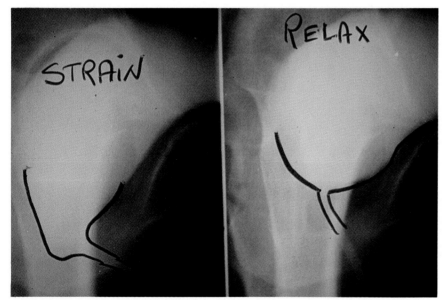

FIGURE 4—7. Lateral relaxed and straining cystogram in a patient with recurrent anatomic stress incontinence after a failed bladder neck suspension operation. The bladder base and urethra are hypermobile due to the loss of support and fixation.

SURGICAL THERAPY

FOR URINARY

INCONTINENCE

A. TRANSVAGINAL NEEDLE BLADDER NECK SUSPENSION

Indications

The most common indication for transvaginal bladder neck suspension (BNS) is anatomic stress incontinence with minimal-to-mild urethral and bladder neck hypermobility. BNS may be performed in conjunction with urethrolysis obstruction, vaginal hysterectomy, repair of urinary fistula, or urethral diverticula.

Contraindications

BNS is not advised in cases of clinical, urodynamic, or radiologic evidence of intrinsic sphincter damage. In cases of moderate or severe cystocele, BNS alone is contraindicated, because it can lead to obstruction or worsening of the cystocele. Detrusor instability is not a contraindication for surgery if genuine stress incontinence can be demonstrated.

Diagnosis

On physical examination with a full bladder, incontinence is objectively demonstrated only on coughing or straining. The incontinence disappears on elevation of the bladder neck, and the urethra and bladder neck are hypermobile. Cystoscopy reveals a hypermobile urethra with posterior-inferior rotation and funneling of the bladder neck upon stress.

Pressure flow studies can be used to confirm the diagnosis in cases of mixed incontinence or prior failure. Patients with anatomic stress incontinence demonstrate leakage of urine without change in the true detrusor pressure.

Video urodynamics show the bladder base relatively well supported, and the urethral axis increased to more than 45 degrees. During stress the bladder neck opens, funnels, and urinary incontinence can be demonstrated with leak pressures above 30 cm H_2O. In the resting-standing position, the bladder neck and urethra are competent.

Preoperative Preparation

The patient is placed in the lithotomy position. The vagina, perineum, and suprapubic area are prepped and draped.

Intraoperative Complications

Urethral bleeding may be avoided by careful dissection over the glistening surface of the periurethral fascia at the level of the bladder neck. Injury to the fascia may require closure of the defect with a small absorbable suture.

Retropubic bleeding may be prevented by entering the retropubic space just at the attachment of the urethropelvic ligament to the lateral pelvic wall. If done more medially, significant bleeding may occur. The suspension sutures will generally stop any bleeding, and extra sutures are rarely applied.

A lower vaginal incision, at the level of the bladder rather than the midurethra, runs the risk of bladder or trigone perforation during the dissection. The inverted U incision, with the apex at the level of the midurethral area, is designed to avoid this complication.

If bladder perforation occurs, it is repaired transvaginally and primarily. A Penrose drain is inserted into the retropubic space and brought to the suprapubic area through a separate incision.

Postoperative Care

Intravenous antibiotics are given for 24 hours, followed by an oral cephalosporin. On the morning after surgery, the urethral catheter, vaginal packing, and intravenous line are discontinued. The suprapubic catheter is plugged, and the patient starts to check the residual urine every 4 hours or as required. Patients are discharged on the first or second day after surgery and may perform normal physical activities (walking, driving, mild lifting) immediately. Sexual intercourse is avoided for 1 month. The suprapubic catheter is removed as soon as the residual of urine is less than 60 ml.

SURGICAL TECHNIQUE

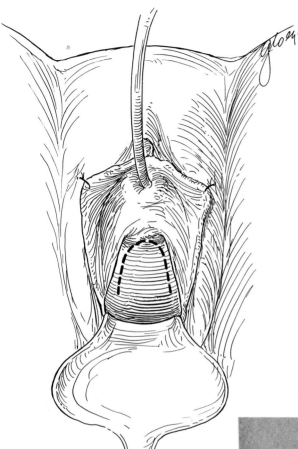

STEP 1:

A weighted speculum is inserted into the vagina, and the labia are sutured to the skin for better exposure. Urethral and suprapubic Number 16 French Foley catheters are inserted. (See Chapter 3, Suprapubic Cystostomy.) The dotted line on the figure indicates the inverted **U** incision of the anterior vaginal wall. (From Walsh PC, Gittes RF, Perlmutter AD, Stamey TA: Campbell Urology, 6th ed. Philadelphia, WB Saunders, 1992.)

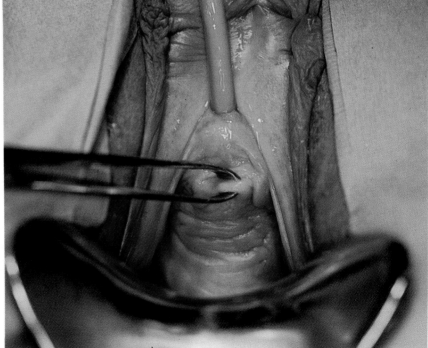

STEP 2:

An Allis clamp grasps the anterior vaginal wall, applying upward traction. It is important that the clamp be placed midway between the bladder neck and the urethral meatus.

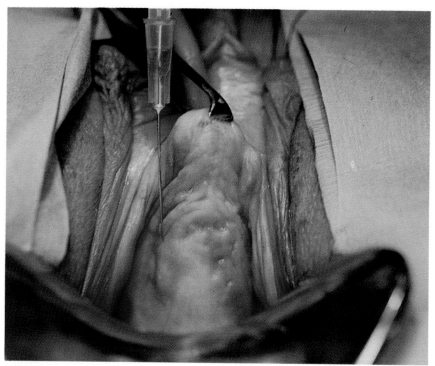

STEP 3:

To facilitate dissection, normal saline (without epinephrine) is injected at the intended line of incision.

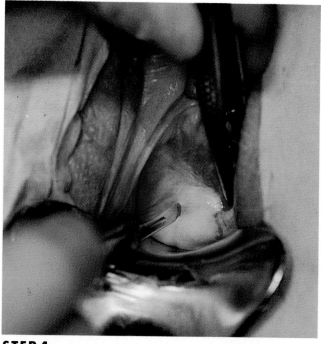

STEP 4:

The anterior vaginal wall is grasped with Bonney forceps, and slight tension is applied to the vaginal wall for better exposure prior to incision.

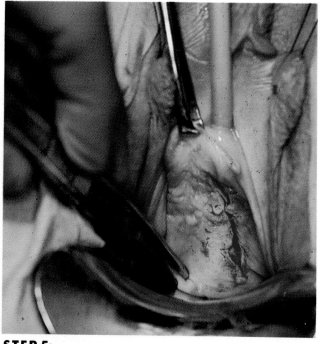

STEP 5:

Two oblique incisions are made in an inverted **U** fashion. Starting in the bladder neck area, the incisions are directed toward the Allis clamp (mid-distance between bladder neck and external meatus). The incisions need not necessarily form a complete **U**.

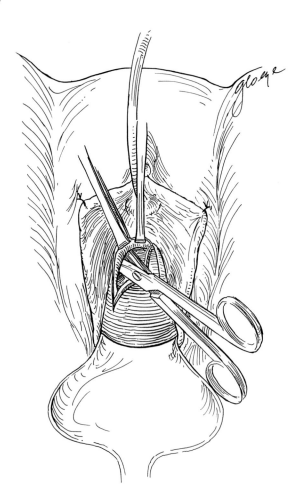

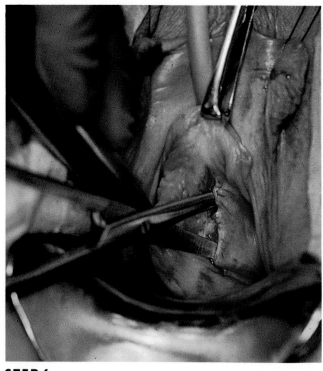

STEP 6:

Using the forceps to grasp the vaginal wall, superficial dissection is carried out over the glistening surface of the periurethral fascia toward the pubic bone. (Drawing from Walsh PC, Gittes RF, Perlmutter AD, Stamey TD: Campbell Urology, 6th ed. Philadelphia, WB Saunders, 1992.)

STEP 7:

With the scissors pointing toward the shoulder of the patient and at the level of the bladder neck, the retropubic space is entered. It is important that the dissection and penetration into the retropubic space be carried out at the level of the urethra. If it is performed at the perivesical level, there is increased risk of bladder penetration and damage.

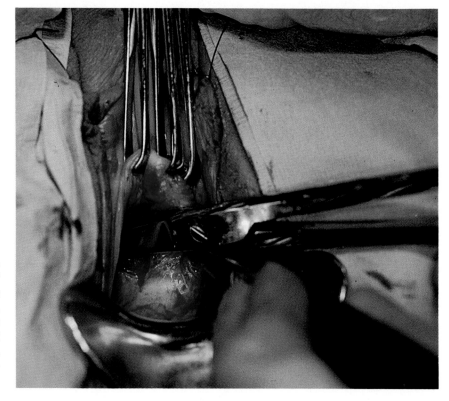

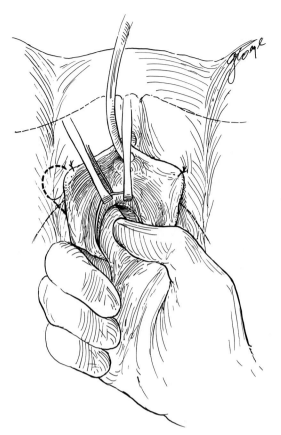

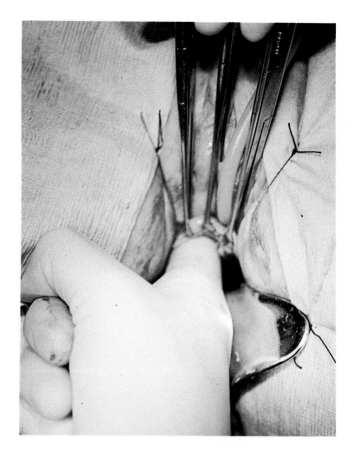

STEP 8:

The urethropelvic ligament is detached from the lateral pelvic wall (tendinous arc).

Adhesions are freed using either sharp or blunt dissection. The anterior vaginal wall is freed between the midurethral area (pubourethral ligament) and the bladder neck. For a successful operation, particularly in patients with prior operations, the anterior vaginal wall should be free of adhesions. If required, a Deaver retractor may be placed in the retropubic space, and sharp dissection under vision can be used to safely incise any urethal adhesions from the pubic bone.

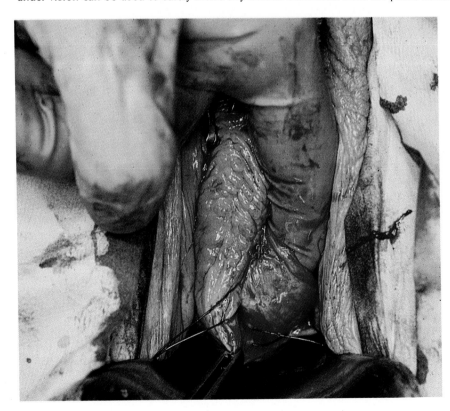

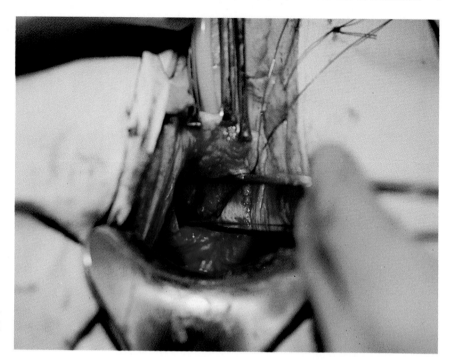

STEP 9:

A long forceps is inserted into the retropubic space and the urethra displaced
medially.

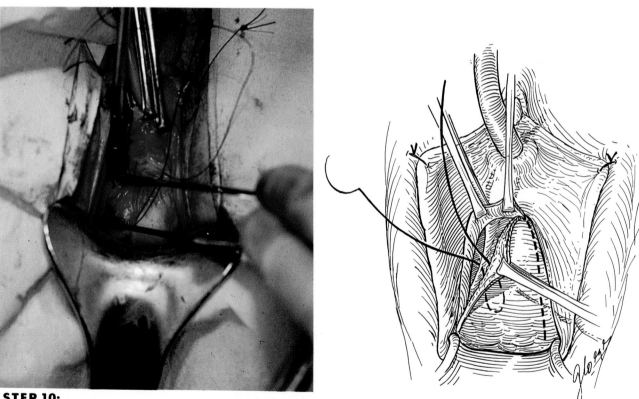

STEP 10:

Number 1 nonabsorbent monofilament sutures (Prolene M0-5 or M0-6 by Ethicon or T-40 Novafil by Davis and Geck) are used to
anchor the medial edge of the urethropelvic ligament, the pubocervical fascia, and the whole vaginal wall except the epithelium.
After three or four helical passes over these structures, the strength of the anchor is tested by pulling the sutures. (One must be able
actually to move the patient.) (Drawing from Walsh PC, Gittes RF, Perlmutter AD, Stamey TA: Campbell Urology, 6th ed.
Philadelphia, WB Saunders, 1992.)

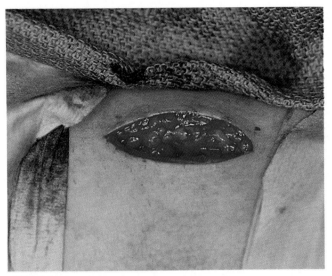

STEP 11:

A 1–2 cm incision is made in the midline, just above the superior margin of the pubic bone, down to the fascia. A higher incision is not recommended because tying the suspending sutures over a mobile area of the anterior abdominal fascia may lead to pain and incomplete support.

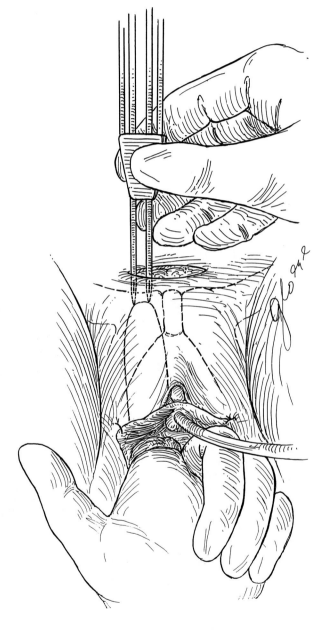

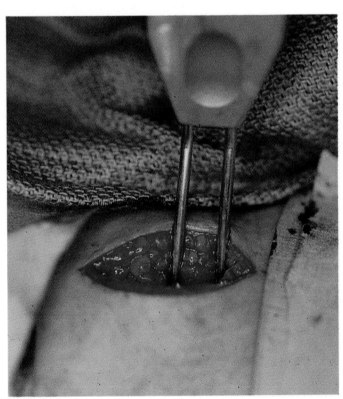

STEP 12:

Using the finger as a guide, a double-pronged ligature carrier (Raz ligature carrier, Cook Company) is transferred from the suprapubic to the vaginal area, as close to the midline and the pubic symphysis as possible; the fascia is thick and less mobile at this point. The ends of the suspending sutures are threaded through the needle holes, and the ligature carrier is pulled upward, bringing the vaginal sutures to the suprapubic incision. The same maneuver is repeated on the other side, with a clamp securing each suture. (Drawing from Walsh PC, Gittes RF, Perlmutter AD, Stamey TA: Campbell Urology, 6th ed. Philadelphia, WB Saunders, 1992.)

STEP 13:

Indigo carmine is injected intravenously, and cystoscopy is performed with 30- and 70-degree optics. This ensures that there is no bladder perforation, the suprapubic catheter is in place, the ureteric excretion of indigo carmine is present in both sides, and, most importantly, the bladder neck and urethra are elevated to a high retropubic position. Upon elevation of the suspending sutures, the bladder neck and urethra should coapt properly.

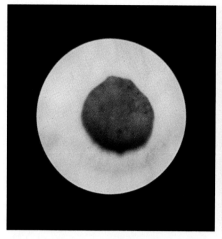
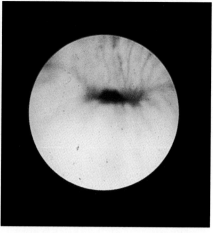

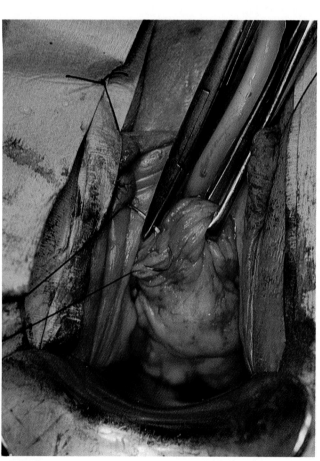
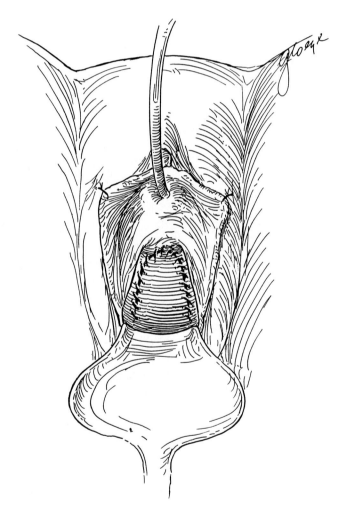

STEP 14:

The anterior vaginal wall is closed with an absorbable running suture of 2-0 polyglycolic acid. A packing laden with antibiotic cream (Sultrim or Betadine) is inserted in the vagina. (Drawing from Walsh PC, Gittes RF, Perlmutter AD, Stamey TA: Campbell Urology, 6th ed. Philadelphia, WB Saunders, 1992.)

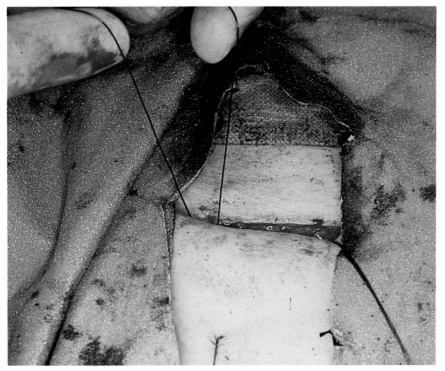

STEP 15:

The Prolene sutures are tied independently on each side over the abdominal fascia and then tied to one another at the midline. If a single-pronged needle is used, the sutures must be tied with a free needle over the fascia or to the pubic bone. The skin is closed with intradermic 4-0 absorbable sutures and Steri-strips.

Postoperative Complications

Delayed vaginal bleeding can be controlled by vaginal packing and bed rest. In cases of excessive bleeding, a Foley catheter with 50 to 80 ml of fluid in the balloon can be inserted posterior to the packing to help control bleeding. Persistent bleeding may require surgical exploration, but so far no patients have required this procedure.

Pain is rare after this operation. Excessive tension of the suspending sutures may lead to prolonged pain, therefore the sutures should not be tightly tied. Other potential sources of suprapubic pain are entrapment of subcutaneous tissue over the fascia and high position of the sutures (the closer they are to the pubic bone, in a nonmobile area, the less pain a patient experiences). The sutures should be applied as close to the midline as possible. Lateral placement may produce persistent pain in the ilioinguinal area.

Permanent urinary retention in a patient with normal bladder function prior to operation is extremely rare. The lateral placement of the sutures (as in the Burch suspension) leaves the urethra free and unobstructed in the retropubic space. If retention is still present 6 months after operation, suprapubic removal under local anesthesia of one or both of the suspending sutures should restart normal voiding.

B. FOUR CORNER BLADDER AND URETHRAL SUSPENSION FOR MODERATE CYSTOCELE

Indications

The goal of this four corner procedure is suspension of the bladder neck and base to correct symptomatic Grade II to III cystocele in patients with mainly paravaginal (lateral) cystocele defect. This procedure may be used with vaginal hysterectomy, enterocele, or rectocele repair.

Contraindications

The presence of Grade IV cystocele is a contraindication for this operation, because of the possibility of further bladder herniation between the suspending sutures. Stress incontinence patients with minimal urethral and bladder neck hypermobility are not good candidates for this operation.

Diagnosis

The main symptoms of moderate cystocele include an anterior vaginal mass, vaginal pressure, stress incontinence, urinary obstruction symptoms, a large residual of urine, and recurrent infections.

During physical examination with a full bladder, the patient is asked to cough or strain. If incontinence is present, it occurs only at the time of stress and disappears on elevation of the bladder neck. The bladder base is hypermobile and reaches to or outside the introitus on straining (Grades II and III, respectively).

Generally, the bladder neck and urethra are also hypermobile, as cystoscopy can confirm. Pressure flow studies are indicated if obstruction, instability, or stress incontinence is present. A VCUG shows the bladder base extending below the inferior rami of the symphysis on straining.

Preoperative Considerations

This operation is an extension of the bladder neck suspension, described in the preceding section. The patient is placed in the lithotomy position and a suprapubic catheter and a weighted vaginal speculum are inserted. In cases of combined hysterectomy and moderate cystocele, the hysterectomy should be performed first, the vaginal cuff closed, and the suspension procedure started.

SURGICAL TECHNIQUE

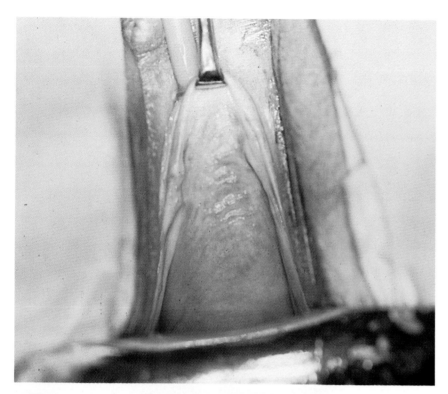

STEP 1:

An Allis clamp grasps the anterior vaginal wall midway between the bladder neck and the urethral meatus, applying upward traction. Normal saline is injected into the anterior vaginal wall at the area of the intended incision.

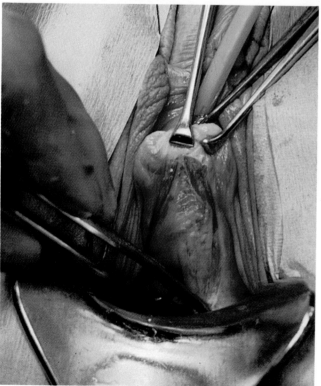

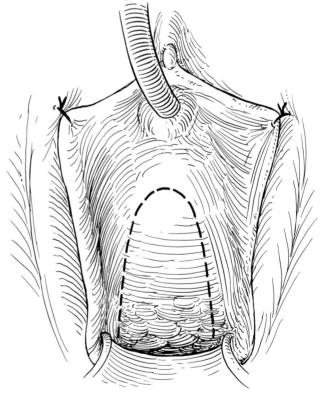

STEP 2:

Two oblique incisions are made in the anterior vaginal wall to form an inverted **U**. The top of the **U** falls midway between the bladder neck and the external meatus, and the legs extend to the cardinal ligaments at the bladder base. If the uterus is present, the incision extends to the paracervical area on each side.

STEP 2 (*continued*):

As in the simple needle bladder neck suspension, the dissection is carried out laterally over the glistening surface of the periurethral fascia. With scissors pointing toward the patient's shoulder, the retropubic space is entered at the level of the bladder neck. It is important to carry the dissection around the midurethral and bladder neck area to minimize chances of bladder performation. At the level of the bladder base the dissection is carried out laterally toward the pubocervical fascia without entering the retropubic space.

STEP 3:

The anterior vaginal wall is freed in the retropubic space between the midurethral area and the bladder neck. Mobilization of the anterior vaginal wall is particularly important in patients previously operated on.

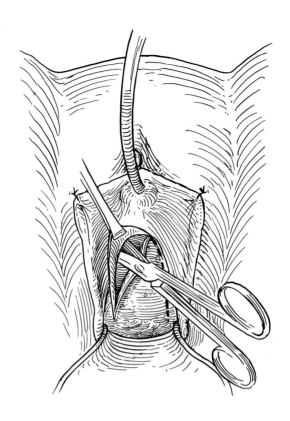

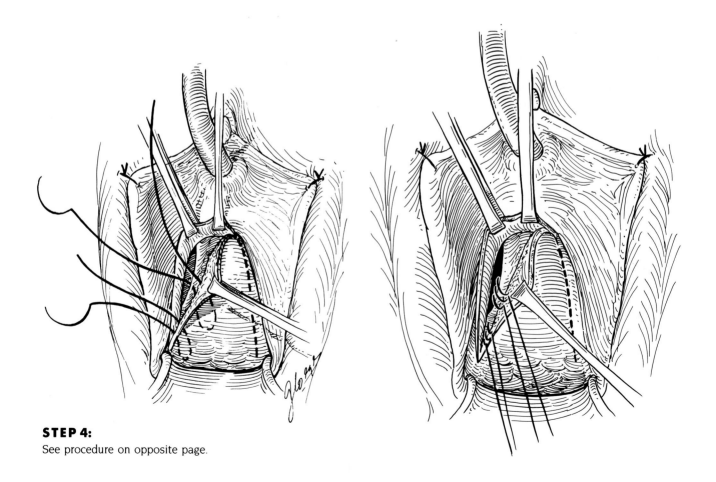

STEP 4:

See procedure on opposite page.

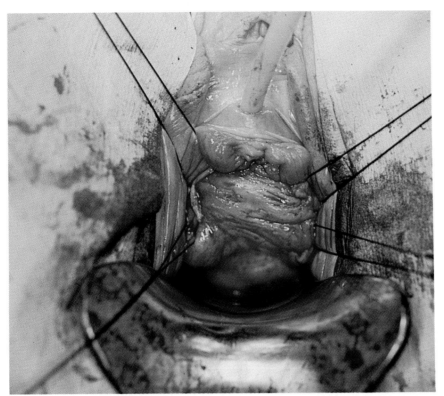

STEP 4:

The bladder and urethra are suspended, using two pairs of Number 1 monofilament nonabsorbable sutures (M0-5 or M0-6 Prolene by Ethicon).

The first pair of sutures is applied at the level of the bladder neck (as described in the preceding section of this chapter). Three or four helicoidal passes of the needle anchor the vaginal wall (without the epithelium), the pubocervical fascia, and, most importantly, the medial edge of the urethropelvic ligament. The strength of the anchor is tested by pulling from the sutures.

The proximal sutures are placed at the base of the inverted **U** incision. These sutures incorporate the vaginal wall (without epithelium), the pubocervical fascia, and the anterior extension of the cardinal ligaments. If the uterus is present, the sutures are applied in the paracervical area on each side. At this point, 5 ml of indigo carmine are injected intravenously.

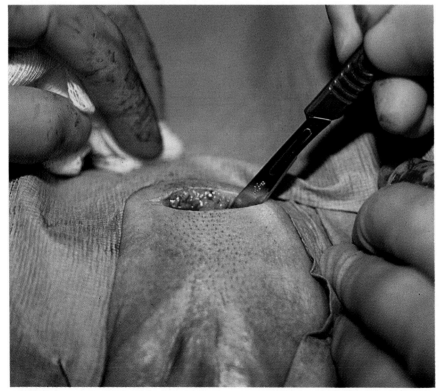

STEP 5:

A 1–2 cm incision is made in the midline, just above the superior margin of the pubic bone. The suspension sutures should be placed at a relatively fixed area of the anterior abdominal wall. An incision over a mobile area of the anterior abdominal fascia may lead to pain and incomplete support.

STEP 6:

Under finger control in the retropubic space, a double-prong ligature carrier is guided from the suprapubic to the vaginal area. The ends of the suspending sutures are passed sequentially through the needle holes, and the ligature carrier is pulled upward to transfer the vaginal sutures to the suprapubic incision. Four passes of the ligature carrier are required. A clamp secures each suture. When the suspending sutures are pulled upward, the anterior vaginal wall and urethra should elevate to a high retropubic position without undue tension on the sutures.

STEP 8:

Cystoscopy is performed with 30- and 70-degree optics to confirm the position of the suprapubic catheter and to rule out bladder perforation and ureter injury. When the suspending sutures are lifted upward, the bladder neck should close properly.

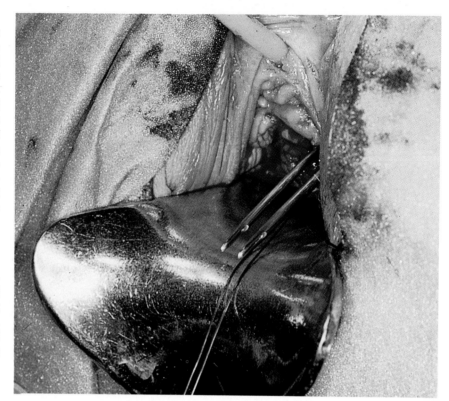

STEP 9:

The anterior vaginal wall is closed with an absorbable running suture of 2-0 Vicryl. A vaginal packing with antibiotic cream (Sultrim or Betadine) is inserted in the vagina. The suspending sutures are tied independently on each side, with multiple knots over the abdominal fascia and then between at the midline. The skin is closed with intradermic 4-0 absorbable sutures and Steri-strips.

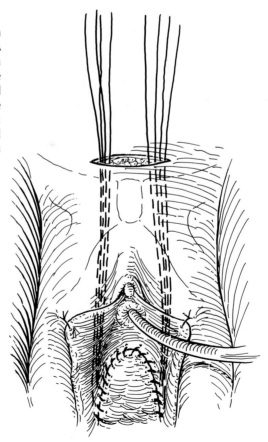

Intraoperative Complications

Potential complications at operation include bleeding, urethra or bladder perforation, and ureteric obstruction from suture malplacement. Lateral dissection over the glistening surface of the periurethral fascia will allow a generally bloodless field. Significant bleeding may occur if the periurethral fascia is perforated or incised. Entering the retropubic space is bloodless if done just at the attachment of the fascia to the pubic bone. The suspension sutures will generally stop any bleeding and rarely are extra sutures applied. A low vaginal incision at the level of the bladder neck rather than at the midurethra risks perforation of the bladder or trigone. The inverted U incision with the apex at the level of the midurethral area is designed to avoid this complication.

Postoperative Care

Intravenous antibiotics are given for 24 hours after operation, followed by oral cephalosporins. Twelve to twenty-four hours after surgery, the urethral catheter, the vaginal packing, and the intravenous line are discontinued. The suprapubic catheter is plugged, and the patient is instructed to check the residual of urine every 4 hours or as required. Patients are discharged 1 or 2 days after surgery.

Postoperative Complications

The most important immediate complications are vaginal bleeding, pain, and prolonged urinary retention. Vaginal bleeding generally stops after tying of the suspending sutures and insertion of the vaginal packing. When excessive bleeding occurs, a large Foley catheter with 50 to 80 ml of fluid in the balloon may be inserted posterior to the packing. Pain after operation is rare and is present mainly in the suprapubic area. The reasons for this pain include tightness of the suprapubic knots, high positioning of the sutures in the suprapubic area, and entrapment of subcutaneous tissue over the fascia. Tying the sutures tightly will lead to pain, not urinary retention. The sutures should not be tied with excessive tension. Permanent urinary retention is extremely unusual, because the lateral placement of the sutures (as in the Burch suspension) leaves the urethra free and unobstructed in the retropubic space. If retention is still present 6 months after operation, removal of one or two of the suspending sutures under local anesthesia should restart normal voiding.

C. SURGICAL REPAIR OF SEVERE ANTERIOR VAGINAL WALL PROLAPSE

Indications

In Grade IV prolapse, the bladder extends outside the introitus at rest. A large cystocele arises, caused by severe weakness of the pubocervical fascia and levator support. Three types of cystocele may be described, depending on the main anatomic defect: (1) a central cystocele, (2) a lateral or paravaginal cystocele, and (3) a combination of both, which is the most common. In central cystocele, the pubocervical fascia and urethropelvic ligaments are still relatively well supported to the lateral pelvic wall, but a central weakness of the pubocervical fascia allows the bladder to prolapse in the center. In lateral cystocele, a weak attachment of the pubocervical fascia and urethropelvic ligament to the lateral pelvic wall allows the whole bladder base to slide downward as a unit.

Cystocele is generally present with concomitant bladder neck and urethral hypermobility (urethrocele). Only on rare occasions, such as after a previous failed operation, may bladder herniation occur without urethral prolapse.

Our transvaginal technique not only repairs the central hernia defect but also simultaneously provides attachment, with nonabsorbable sutures, of the bladder neck and base, including pubocervical and cardinal ligaments, to the pubic bone for support, thus avoiding paravaginal or lateral sliding of the bladder wall. Should one repair only the central defect, the cystocele may recur owing to the lack of lateral support, and de novo incontinence may ensue because of a poorly supported and hypermobile urethra, now in a low dependent position. On the other hand, if only a bladder neck suspension is performed without correction of the cystocele, the patient may develop aggravation of the prolapse, obstructive symptoms, and urinary retention.

In general, Grade IV prolapse is present in conjunction with other anatomic abnormalities, including uterine prolapse, enterocele (in posthysterectomy patients), rectocele, or vaginal vault prolapse. These conditions, discussed in separate sections, should be corrected at the time of cystocele repair.

Indications for operation include a symptomatic mass always outside the vagina; urinary incontinence with Grade IV cystocele; voiding dysfunction, including obstruction, frequency, and urgency; large postvoid residuals; and recurrent urinary tract infections.

Diagnosis

The patient generally senses a bulging mass through the introitus, with or without stress urinary incontinence. On physical examination with a full bladder, the bladder base is seen bulging through the introitus at rest. An increase in the protrusion can be detected when the patient coughs or strains.

Cystoscopy may show hypermobility and funneling of the bladder neck and marked descent of the bladder base and trigone.

Radiologic studies (VCUG) and video urodynamics (Fig. 5-1) show the bladder base to have descended well beyond the inferior rami of the symphysis. The bladder neck may be funneled, and stress-induced urinary incontinence may be present. During straining the cystocele is further enlarged. Commonly patients void normally with low residuals, but some patients, particularly those after previous operation, may show an obstructive pattern and an increase in postvoid urinary residual. Intravenous pyelogram or a kidney ultrasound study is indicated to rule out partial ureteral obstruction or hydronephrosis.

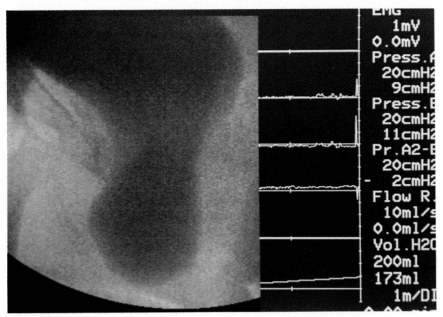

FIGURE 5–1. Standing video urodynamics and cystogram in a patient with Grade IV cystocele. No incontinence is demonstrated.

SURGICAL TECHNIQUE

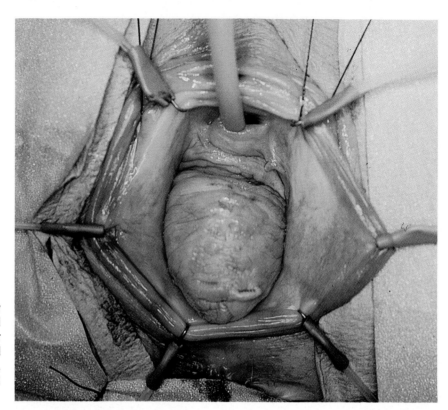

STEP 1:

With the patient in the dorsal lithotomy position, a suprapubic cystostomy and urethral catheter are inserted. The bladder is emptied. A Scott retractor is positioned and secured with 6 hooks in the upper, medial, and lower thirds of the vaginal introitus.

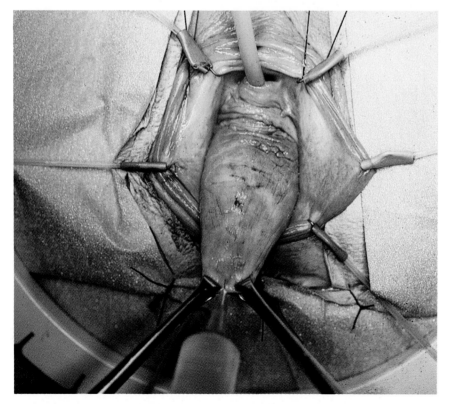

STEP 2:

Using Allis clamps to expose the vaginal wall. Normal saline is injected to facilitate the dissection.

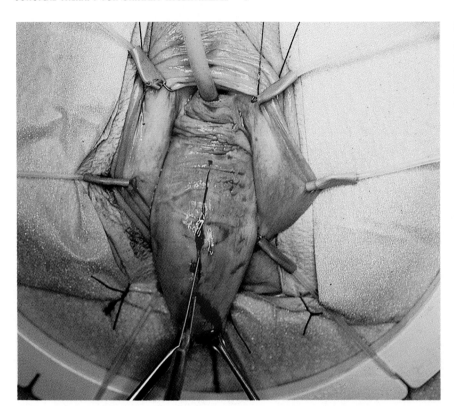

STEP 3:

A vertical incision is made, extending from the midurethra down to the bladder base. (Drawing from Walsh PC, Gittes RF, Perlmutter AD, Stamey TA: Campbell Urology, 6th ed. Philadelphia, WB Saunders, 1992.)

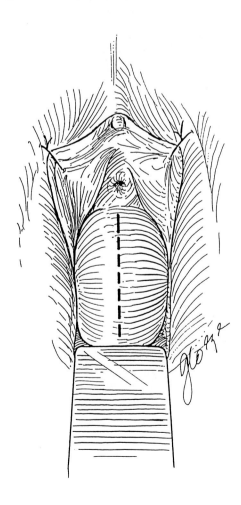

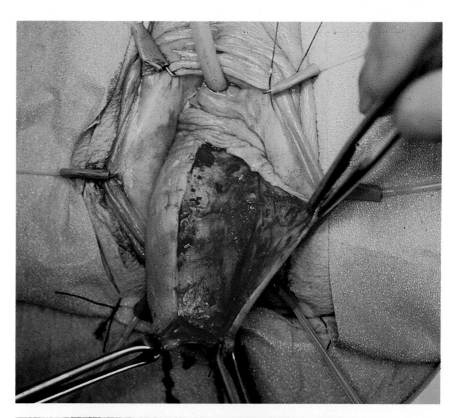

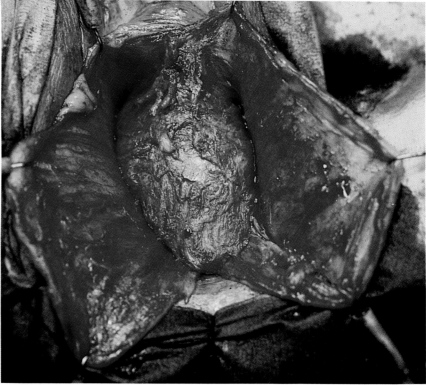

STEP 4:

The dissection is carried out in the avascular plane between the vaginal wall and the bladder (vesicovaginal space), laterally toward the pubocervical fascia. By keeping a superficial dissection, bladder injury should be avoided.

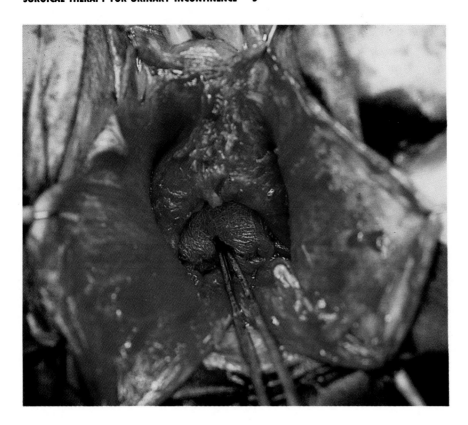

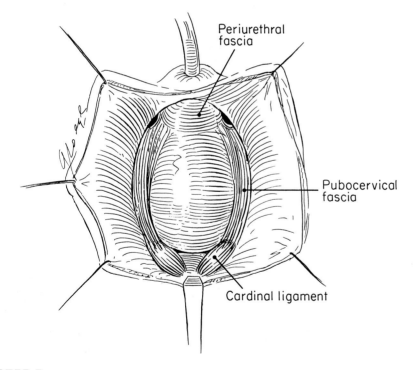

Periurethral
fascia

Pubocervical
fascia

Cardinal ligament

STEP 5:

The lateral dissection exposes the pubocervical fascia in the sides and the periurethral fascia and attenuated cardinal ligaments at the bladder base. A folded gauze is used to reduce the cystocele and further demonstrate the medial edge of the pubocervical fascia. Posteriorly, the dissection will reach the peritoneal fold. If indicated, hysterectomy or enterocele repair should be performed at this stage of the operation. (Drawing from Walsh PC, Gittes RF, Perlmutter AD, Stamey TA: Campbell Urology, 6th ed. Philadelphia, WB Saunders, 1992.)

STEP 6:

Dissecting over the glistening surface of the periurethral fascia, toward the pubic bone, the urethropelvic ligaments are detached from the tendinous arc. The retropubic space is entered on each side, and all adhesions are dissected free. A finger in the retropubic space demonstrates the medial edge of the urethropelvic ligaments.

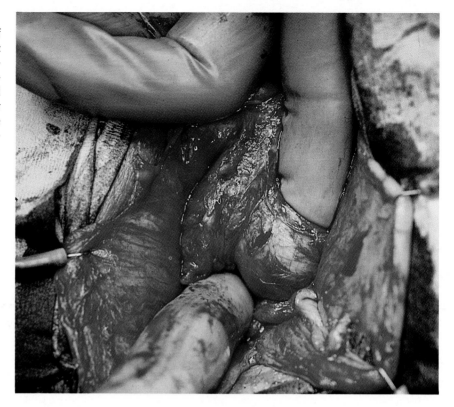

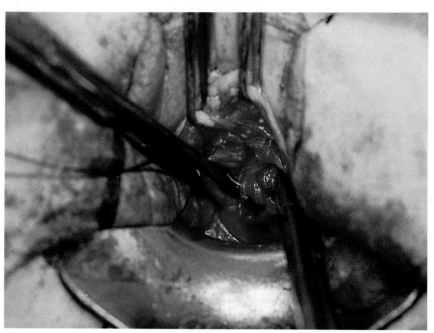

STEP 7:

Number 1 Prolene sutures are applied bilaterally in a helical fashion to include the vaginal wall (without epithelium), the medial edge of the detached urethropelvic ligaments, and the pubocervical fascia, extending to the anterior portion of the cardinal ligaments. The distance between these structures is generally no more than 2 to 3 cm, but if it is larger than 3 cm we will apply 4 Prolene sutures (two at the bladder neck and two at the bladder base to include pubocervical and cardinal ligaments). The goal of these sutures is to provide good lateral support to the bladder neck and bladder base (paravaginal defect).

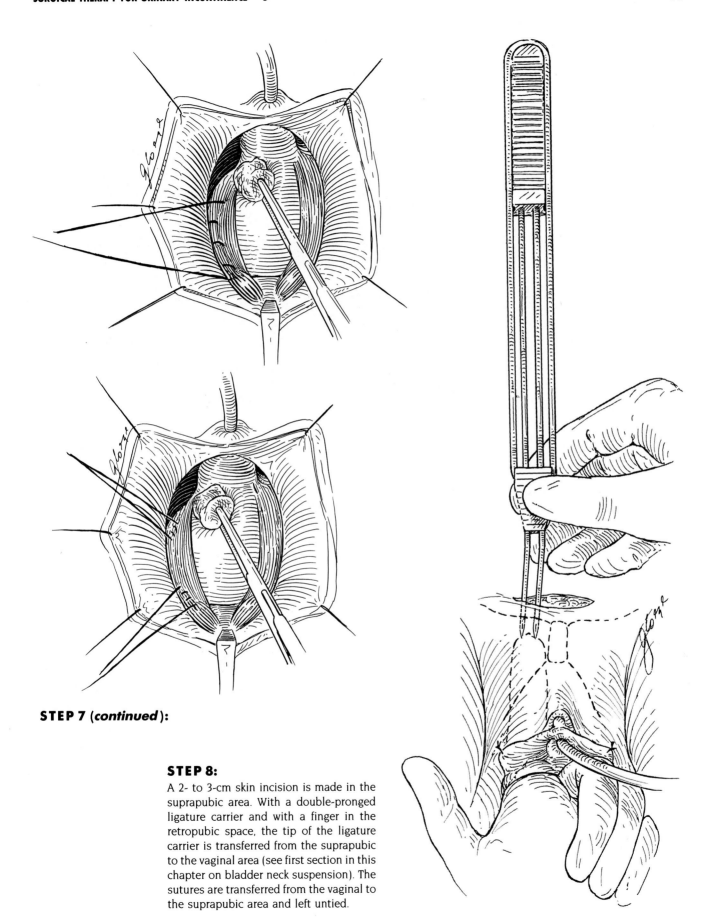

STEP 7 (*continued*):

STEP 8:

A 2- to 3-cm skin incision is made in the suprapubic area. With a double-pronged ligature carrier and with a finger in the retropubic space, the tip of the ligature carrier is transferred from the suprapubic to the vaginal area (see first section in this chapter on bladder neck suspension). The sutures are transferred from the vaginal to the suprapubic area and left untied.

STEP 9:

Interrupted figure eight 2-0 Vicryl sutures are applied from the bladder neck to bladder base, approximating the medial edge of the pubocervical fascia. An important step is the approximation of the cardinal ligaments at the bladder base. This maneuver will reconstruct the rectangular plate supporting the bladder base. The vaginal wall is not included in the suture line.

At the level of the vaginal cuff the cardinal ligaments are identified, anchored, and approximated to the midline. This important step provides further strength to the repair of the herniated bladder, narrowing the gap between the laterally displaced pubocervical fasciae. The photograph shows the completion of this step, with the prolene sutures providing the lateral support (the anchoring of the pubocervical fascia, cardinal ligaments, and bladder neck), and the approximation of the pubocervical fascia correcting the central defect.

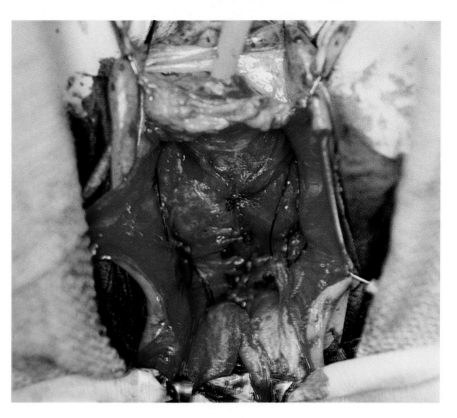

STEP 10:

Indigo carmine is administered intravenously, and cystoscopy is performed. This test will confirm proper positioning of the suprapubic tube, adequate efflux of dye from the ureteral orifices, and the absence of bladder injury. Adequate closure and support of the bladder neck and proximal urethra should be observed with gentle traction on the suspension sutures.

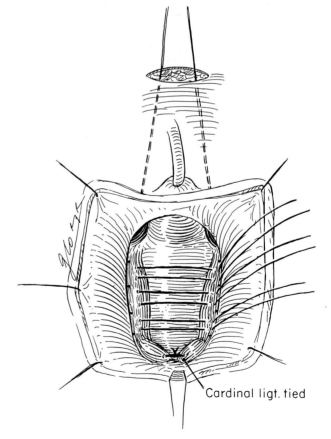

Cardinal ligt. tied

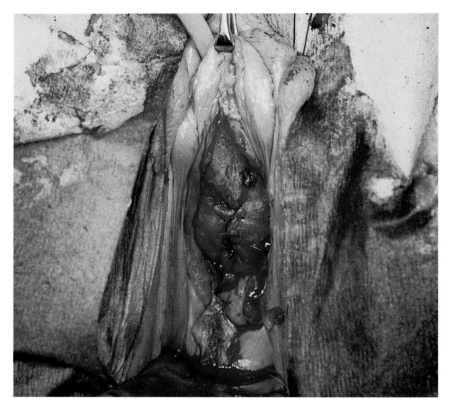

STEP 11:

The excess vaginal wall is trimmed and excised. The vaginal incision is closed with a running 2-0 Vicryl suture, incorporating the underlying pubocervical fascia to eliminate any "dead space." A vaginal packing coated with antibiotic cream is inserted.

STEP 12:

The suspension sutures are tied in the suprapubic space, individually and then to one another across the midline. The suprapubic incision is closed with a running subcuticular 4-0 Dexon suture.

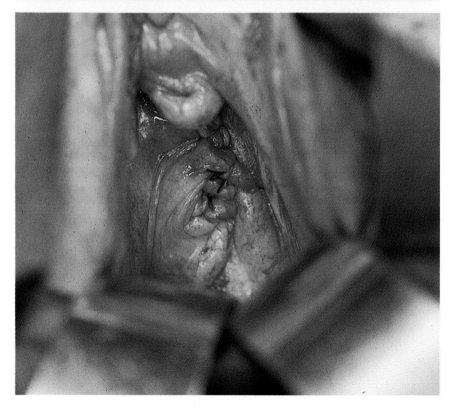

Intraoperative Complications

As in other vaginal procedures, the potential complications during surgery include bleeding, urethra or bladder perforation, and ureteric obstruction. In this operation special attention should be given to the ureters because of their close proximity to the surgical repair. The bladder and trigone should be retracted above the level of the pelvic floor when placing the midline sutures over the pubocervical fascia. Cystoscopy should confirm the patency of both ureteric orifices; when this is in doubt, a stent should be inserted. If ureter obstruction is found, the suspension or pubocervical fascia sutures should be removed and replaced.

Bladder injury at the time of dissection should be repaired primarily, using a multiple layer of delayed absorbable sutures and prolonged bladder drainage. With anterior bladder injury, a Penrose drain may be inserted in the retropubic space, using a percutaneous technique.

Postoperative Care

The vaginal packing and urethral catheter are removed 24 hours after operation. The suprapubic catheter is plugged, and the patient checks the residuals every 4 hours or as required.

Postoperative Complications

Postoperative complications are similar to those of other vaginal reconstructive procedures. Prolonged urinary retention is rare and is managed by leaving the suprapubic tube indwelling for a longer period of time. If the problem persists after a month, the patient is started on a self–intermittent catheterization program until adequate bladder emptying resumes.

De novo or recurrent stress incontinence may develop as a result of inadequate support of the bladder neck and urethra (anatomic incontinence) or because of an open, incompetent, nonfunctional proximal sphincteric area (intrinsic sphincter dysfunction).

Recurrent prolapse of the bladder is very rare and may result from inappropriate positioning of the sutures or from poor quality of tissues, in particular when severe atrophic vaginitis is present.

In patients with Grade IV cystocele, concomitant surgical procedures such as hysterectomy and enterocele and rectocele repair are required in more than 75 per cent of cases. Repair of the cystocele without repair of these abnormalities may lead to their further aggravation, requiring another operation. Secondary enterocele or rectocele may occur. The transfer of the anterior vaginal wall to a high supported position may bring about a weakened cul de sac and cause the posterior vaginal wall to herniate.

Vaginal shortening may occur if excess vaginal wall is removed. Bearing in mind the concept of this operation as a bladder suspension, very little vaginal tissue is excised, and this complication can be avoided.

Pain in the suprapubic area is rare and may result from nerve entrapment, passage of the suspending sutures higher than the superior margin of the symphysis (mobile portion of the abdominal wall), tight knots, or a low-grade infection.

Ureter obstruction after operation, despite cystoscopic patency at the time of operation, results from kinking of the ureters by the suspending sutures. A percutaneous nephrostomy should be inserted if endoscopic passage of a guide wire or stent is unsuccessful. After a prudent period of observation, the procedure could be tried again. If it fails, ureter reimplantation may be indicated. We prefer not to explore transvaginally the area of ureter obstruction, to avoid undue damage of an otherwise good anatomic repair.

D. SLING PROCEDURES

Vaginal Wall Sling

Indications

A vaginal wall sling is indicated for patients with urinary incontinence secondary to severe sphincter incompetence. In these cases the urethra is no longer acting as a sphincter unit. Intrinsic sphincter incompetence most often is associated with multiple failed anti-incontinence procedures, resulting in a fixed, open urethra in a normal anatomic position. Other causes are radiation, pelvic fracture, and neuropathic urethral dysfunction. The sling procedure aims at creating a hammock that supports and compresses the urethra, thus resulting in improved coaptation of the urethral walls and continence.

Contraindications

The sling procedure is relatively contraindicated in patients with atrophic vaginitis. In these cases the vaginal wall will not be of sufficient integrity and tensile strength to be used as a sling. If recognized preoperatively, this problem can be circumvented with the administration of vaginal estrogen preparations.

Patients who undergo construction of a sling are at a higher risk of urinary retention, which might necessitate a patient's performing self-intermittent catheterization. The patient should be physically and mentally capable of doing the catheterization.

Diagnosis

The clinical presentation is that of severe positional incontinence, usually with a history of multiple surgical procedures for incontinence or urethral trauma, or as a result of irradiation. The patient complains of gravitational (not associated with stress) urinary leakage in both the upright and sometimes in the supine position. Cystourethroscopy demonstrates a fixed and open bladder neck, and the urethra has the appearance of a "lead pipe," denoting the rigidity and scarring of the urethral wall (Fig. 5–2). A VCUG will demonstrate the severe incontinence, with the bladder neck and urethra open at rest and with stress. Video urodynamics reveal leakage of urine with minimal increase in abdominal pressures during Valsalva maneuvers (in general, leak pressures are less than 30 cm H_2O).

Intraoperative Complications

Potential complications at operation are bleeding, urethra or bladder perforation during the dissection, and ureter obstruction by the suspension sutures.

Postoperative Care

The urethral catheter, vaginal packing, and intravenous line are removed on the day following surgery. The patient is instructed to check postvoid residuals via the suprapubic catheter, and she generally is discharged from the hospital 2 days postoperatively. When spontaneous voiding resumes and the postvoid residuals become negligible, the suprapubic tube is removed in the surgeon's office.

Postoperative Complications

Any sling technique involves risks of delayed voiding, obstructive urinary symptoms, and even permanent urinary retention. However, in our experience less than 5 percent of the patients with non-neurogenic urethral incompetence has suffered from permanent retention. De novo instability causing irritation can occur; this usually responds to anticholinergic medication. Vaginal shortening has not been found to be a problem to date. We have encountered no problems with burying the island of vaginal epithelium; however, we recognize the potential risk of cyst formation.

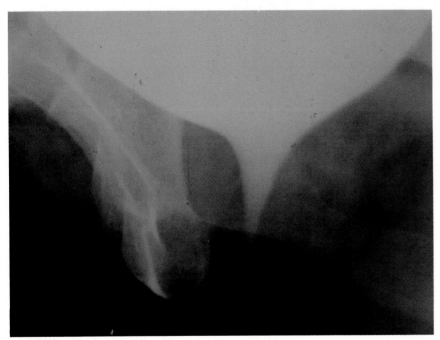

FIGURE 5—2. Standing cystogram in a patient suffering from severe urinary incontinence after many operations. The bladder neck and urethra are open and incompetent.

SURGICAL TECHNIQUE

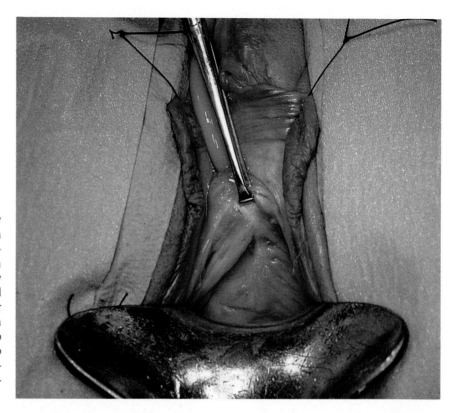

STEP 1:

The patient is placed in a dorsal lithotomy position. The lower abdomen and vagina are prepped and draped in a sterile fashion. The labia are retracted laterally with stay sutures. A suprapubic cystostomy tube is placed via a Lowsley retractor, and a urethral catheter is inserted. The bladder is emptied. A weighted vaginal speculum is placed. An Allis clamp is used to grasp the anterior vaginal wall just proximal to the urethral meatus. Normal saline is injected in the anterior vaginal wall to facilitate the dissection.

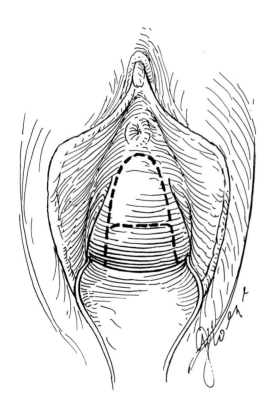

STEP 2:

A complete inverted **U** incision is made, with the apex just proximal to the urethral meatus and the base extended several centimeters proximal to the bladder neck. A second incision is made at the level of the bladder neck to join the two legs of the inverted **U** incision. (From Walsh PC, Gittes RF, Perlmutter AD, Stamey TA: Campbell Urology, 6th ed. Philadelphia, WB Saunders, 1992.)

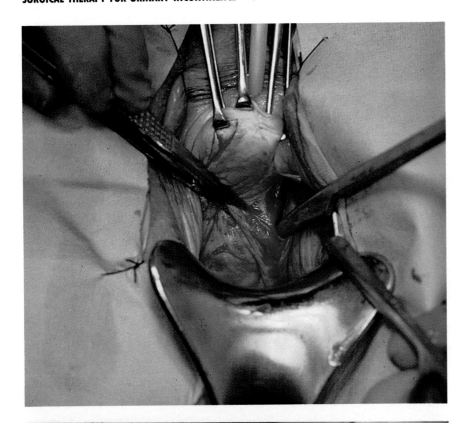

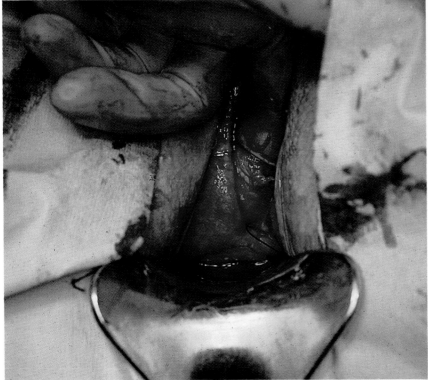

STEP 3:

The vaginal epithelium is dissected laterally along the glistening white periurethral fascia, toward the pubic bone. Sharp and blunt dissection is used to enter the retropubic space. The urethra is mobilized by freeing the lateral attachments of the urethropelvic fascia and all previous adhesions from the level of the pubis to the ischial tuberosity, using blunt and sharp dissection.

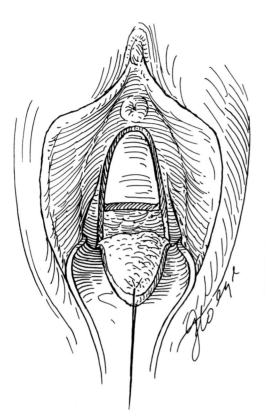
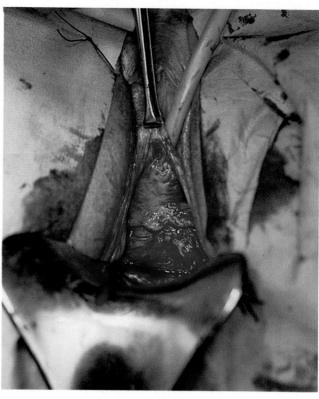

STEP 4:

Starting at the level of the bladder neck, the proximal vaginal wall is dissected to create a pediculated flap of adequate length to cover the urethra in a later step of the operation. This creates a rectangular island of anterior vaginal wall that underlies the bladder neck and urethra, retains its own vascular supply, and will function as the sling. The size of this island is tailored easily to the length and width of the urethra. (Drawing from Walsh PC, Gittes RF, Perlmutter AD, Stamey TA: Campbell Urology, 6th ed. Philadelphia, WB Saunders, 1992.)

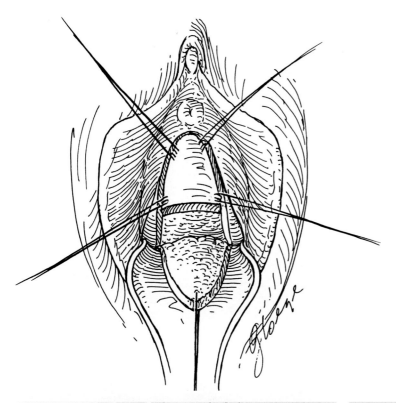

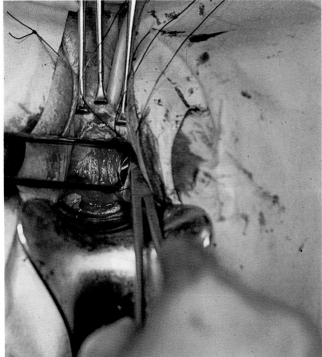

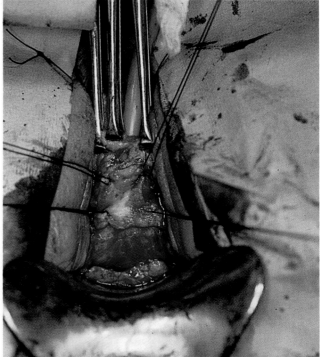

STEP 5:

The four corners of the rectangular island of vaginal wall are anchored with individual sutures of Number 1 Prolene applied in a helical fashion. The two proximal sutures are applied at the level of the bladder neck, incorporating the urethropelvic fascia, pubocervical and periurethral fascia, and full thickness of the proximal corners of the vaginal wall rectangle. The two distal sutures include the periurethral fascia and the distal corners of the sling.

The anchoring strength of these sutures is tested by pulling on the sutures. The vaginal wall itself is not the main anchoring or compressing element of the sling; rather it adds only to the strength of the urethropelvic and periurethral fascia anchors. (Drawing from Walsh PC, Gittes RF, Perlmutter AD, Stamey TA: Campbell Urology, 6th ed. Philadelphia, WB Saunders, 1992.)

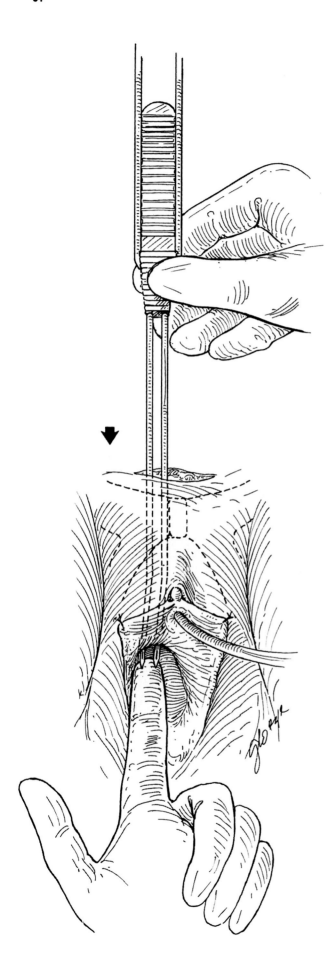

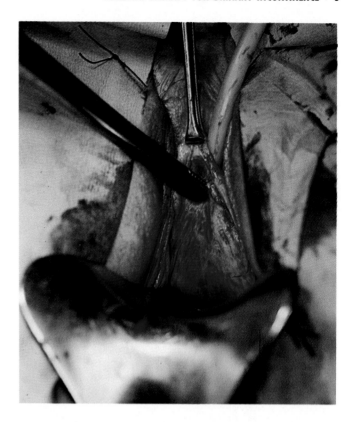

STEP 6:

A small transverse skin incision is made just superior to the pubic symphysis and is extended down to the rectus fascia. A double-pronged ligature carrier is used to transfer the Prolene sutures individually from the vagina to the suprapubic region under finger control. Four passes of the ligature carrier are required. Finger guidance in the retropubic space prevents inadvertent penetration of the bladder and urethra. The double-pronged carrier will permit the sutures to be tied over a 1-cm segment of the rectus fascia.

Five milliliters of indigo carmine are administered intravenously, the urethral catheter is removed, and cystourethroscopy is performed. The goals of the endoscopic examination are (1) to ensure that the urethra and bladder neck are compressed, well coapted, and suspended effectively when minimal traction is placed on the suspension sutures; (2) to confirm that the urethra and bladder have not been penetrated by a suture; (3) to assure proper efflux of urine from the ureteral orifices, and (4) to verify adequate positioning of the suprapubic tube. Following cystoscopy, the urethral catheter is replaced.

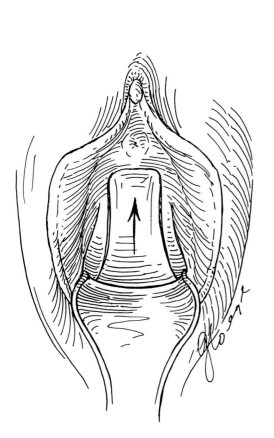

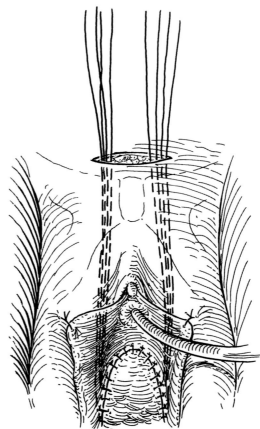

STEP 7:

The proximal vaginal wall flap, previously developed and mobilized, is advanced over the sling to provide an epithelial cover and restore the integrity of the vagina, using a 2-0 absorbable polyglycolic acid suture. (From Walsh PC, Gittes RF, Perlmutter AD, Stamey TA: Campbell Urology, 6th ed. Philadelphia, WB Saunders, 1992.)

STEP 8:

All Prolene sutures are tied individually and then to each other across the midline without undue tension. The suprapubic incision is closed with running subcuticular 4-0 polyglycolic acid suture, and a vaginal packing impregnated with antibiotic cream is placed. The urethral catheters and suprapubic tube are connected to a closed bag drainage.

Pubovaginal Sling

Indications

Construction of a pubovaginal sling is indicated for stress urinary incontinence secondary to intrinsic sphincter damage (type III incontinence). We currently use this procedure when creation of a vaginal wall sling is not feasible due to poor tissue quality. Nevertheless, many surgeons prefer this procedure primarily. From a historical standpoint, several sources for the pubovaginal sling have been utilized, such as pyramidal muscle and fascia, rectus muscle, and fascia lata. The technique we describe herein is based on the rectus fascia, as described by Dr. E. McGuire at the University of Michigan.

Contraindications

Patients who undergo construction of a sling are at risk of developing urinary retention that might necessitate self-intermittent catheterization for a prolonged period of time, sometimes for the rest of their lives. The patient should be aware of such a possibility and needs to be able to perform self-catheterization.

Intraoperative Complications

Potential intraoperative complications include injury to the urethra, bladder, or ureters during the dissection and during transfer of the suspension sutures. Bowel injury may occur during insertion of the suprapubic tube.

Postoperative Care

The Foley catheter and the vaginal packing are removed on the morning following operation. Intravenous antibiotics are given for 24 hours, followed by oral antibiotics for several days. The suprapubic catheter is plugged and the patient unplugs it to empty the bladder or to measure postvoid residuals. When the postvoid residuals dwindle, the suprapubic tube is withdrawn. If after a few weeks the patient is still experiencing retention, she is taught self-intermittent catheterization and the suprapubic tube is removed.

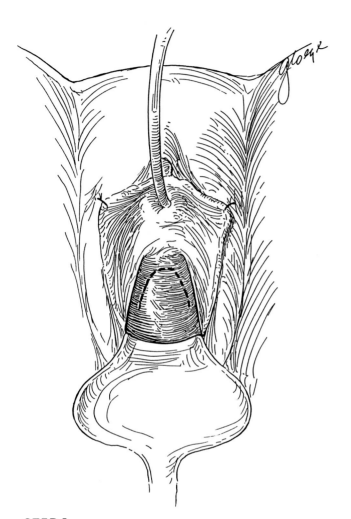

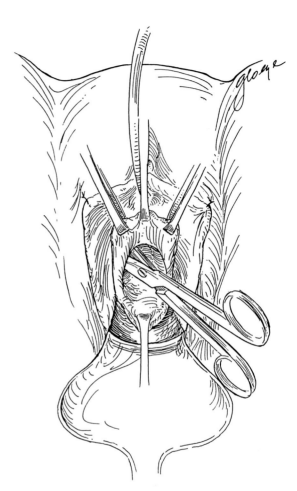

STEP 1:

A combined abdominal-vaginal approach is used for the operation. The patient is placed in the dorsal lithotomy position. The lower abdomen and vagina are prepped and draped in sterile fashion. The labia are retracted laterally with stay sutures. A suprapubic cystostomy tube is placed and a urethral Foley catheter is inserted. The bladder is drained. A weighted posterior vaginal retractor is placed.

With the patient in the lithotomy position, a semicircular incision is made in the anterior vaginal wall. Alternatively, two oblique incisions can be made in the anterior vaginal wall. A tunnel 2 cm wide may be dissected between the vaginal wall and the bladder neck area. The sling can be transferred later through this space, obviating the creation of a vaginal wall flap.

STEP 2:

A flap of vaginal wall is dissected free with its base toward the bladder. Dissection is carried out over the glistening surface of the periurethral area toward the tendinous arc of the obturator muscle. The retropubic space is entered with scissors pointing toward the ipsilateral shoulder of the patient.

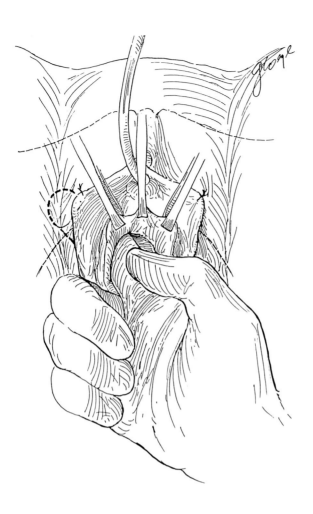

STEP 2 (*continued*):

The retropubic space is freed from adhesions, and a tunnel is created toward the suprapubic area.

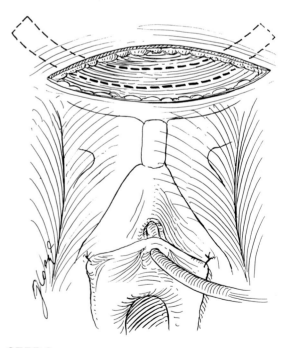

STEP 3:

A transverse incision is made over the suprapubic area, exposing the anterior abdominal fascia. The incision for the retrieval of the fascial graft is outlined.

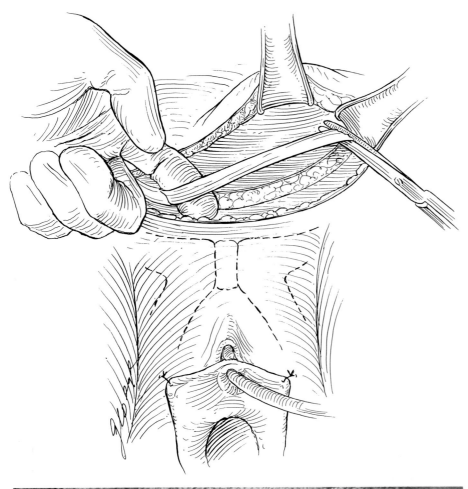

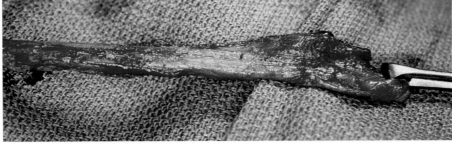

STEP 3 (*continued*):

The strip of fascia is detached from the underlying musculature and incised at the corners.

A transverse fascial flap is created, measuring approximately 2 to 3 cm in width by 12 to 15 cm in length, with the middle segment wider than the edges. The graft is sharply dissected from the underlying rectus muscle. A number 1 Prolene suture is then placed in a helical fashion in each free edge of the fascial strip. The fascial strip is temporarily immersed in normal saline for further use. The fascial defect is closed with interrupted figure eight polyglycolic acid sutures.

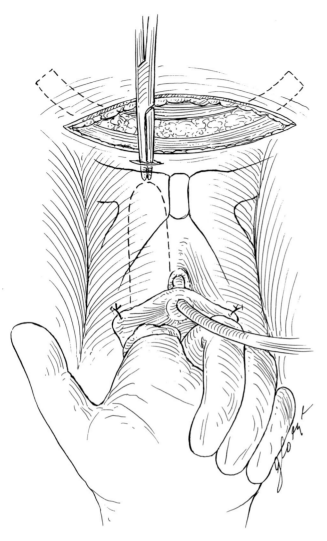

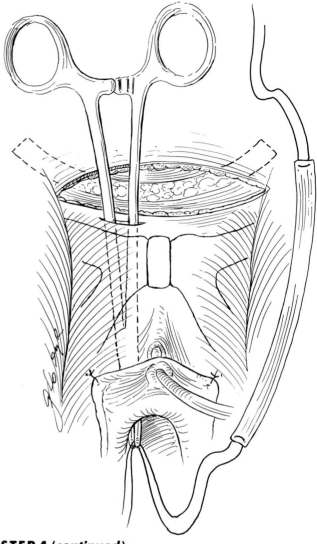

STEP 4:

A 1-cm incision is made just above the pubic bone on each side of the midline, the two incisions being 5 cm apart. A tonsil clamp is passed under finger guidance through the retropubic space and out through the vaginal incision.

STEP 4 (*continued*):

One end of the graft is transferred from the vaginal to the suprapubic area by grasping the anchoring Number 1 Prolene suture. One edge of the Prolene suture is threaded into an empty needle and is secured to the rectus fascia in a helical fashion and then tied to the other edge, thus fixing one side of the sling. The free end of the sling is placed around the urethrovesical junction, and the second pair of Prolene sutures is grasped in the same manner through the contralateral retropubic space and is transferred to the suprapubic position.

STEP 5:

The adequacy of the sling suspension is determined through cystoscopy, which should demonstrate coaptation of the bladder neck with traction on the suspension sutures. The fascial strip is marked for its proper location, but its free end is not secured yet. It is recommended that the fascial strip be anchored to the area of the bladder neck with interrupted absorbable sutures. This will prevent slippage of the sling from the desired point of compression at the bladder neck. Indigo carmine is injected intravenously, and the ureteral orifices are inspected for efflux of dye. Proper positioning of the suprapubic tube is also determined. The cystoscope is removed and the urethral Foley catheter is replaced.

STEP 6:

After closure of the vaginal wall, the end of the sling is anchored to the suprapubic area with the previously placed Prolene sutures. Tension should be avoided.

The abdominal incision is closed and a vaginal packing is placed. Both catheters are connected to a closed bag drainage.

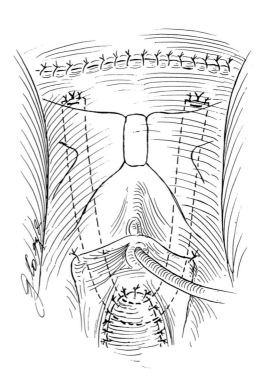

Postoperative Complications

Failure of the sling to cure incontinence can result from inadequate coaptation of the urethra by the compressive sling or secondary to detrusor hyperactivity and urgency incontinence. De novo bladder instability is found in 15 to 20 percent of the cases requiring cholinolytic therapy. Chronic urinary retention, requiring self–intermittent catheterization for a lifetime, is rare but may occur following surgery.

RECTANGULAR FASCIAL SLING: AN ALTERNATIVE METHOD

An alternative method for the construction of a fascial sling is the use of an isolated rectangle of anterior abdominal wall fascia. The surgical steps are similar to those for the pubovaginal sling.

The advantage of this procedure is its simplicity. There is no extensive dissection in the suprapubic area, and the postoperative result is similar to that of the full-length fascial strip sling.

The postoperative care is similar to that of the pubovaginal sling.

E. PERIURETHRAL OR TRANSURETHRAL INJECTION OF TEFLON PASTE

Indications

Patients with urethral related urinary incontinence without a significant anatomic abnormality are candidates for periurethral Teflon (polytetrafluoroethylene) injections. The goal of the surgery is to provide better coaptation and seal to the incompetent urethral mechanism by the cushion effect created by the Teflon paste under the urethral mucosa. Teflon initiates a foreign body reaction and granuloma formation in the injection site. The best candidates for this procedure are patients who have not undergone radiation therapy, are suffering from recurrent stress incontinence after failed operation, and have relatively good anatomic support (Fig. 5–3).

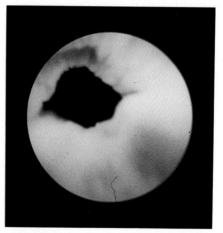

FIGURE 5–3. Urethroscopy of a patient with severe incontinence after multiple surgical procedures. The urethra is well supported but open all the time.

SURGICAL TECHNIQUE

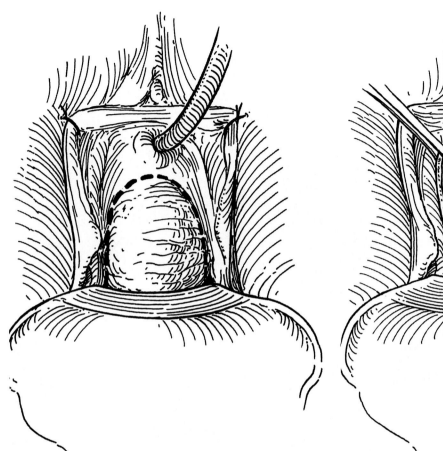

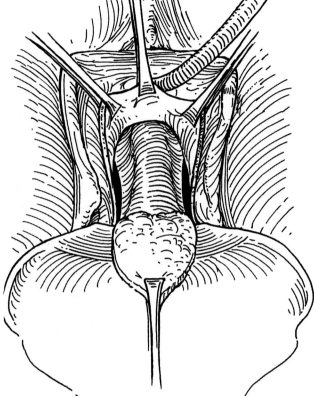

STEP 1:

A semicircular incision is made in the anterior vaginal wall.

STEP 2:

A vaginal wall flap is dissected posteriorly, exposing the periurethral fascia. After entering the retropubic space, sharp and blunt dissection is used to form a tunnel toward the superior rami of the pubic bone.

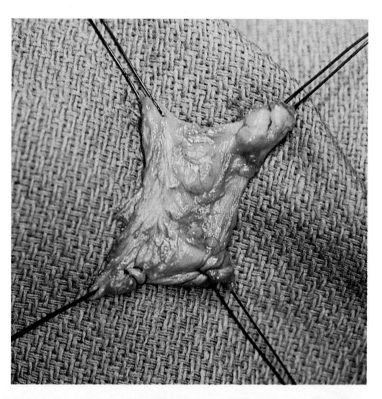

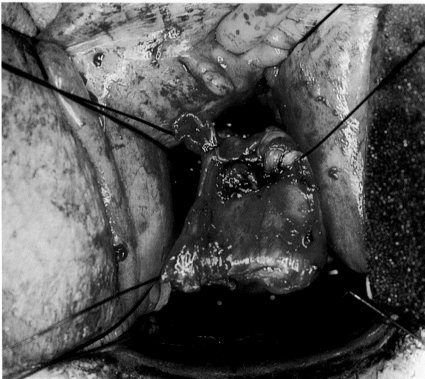

STEP 3:

A small incision is made in the suprapubic area (5 cm in length). A small 3 × 4 cm rectangle of fascia is retrieved and the anterior abdominal wall closed. The four corners of the rectangle are anchored with Number 1 Prolene sutures in a helical fashion.

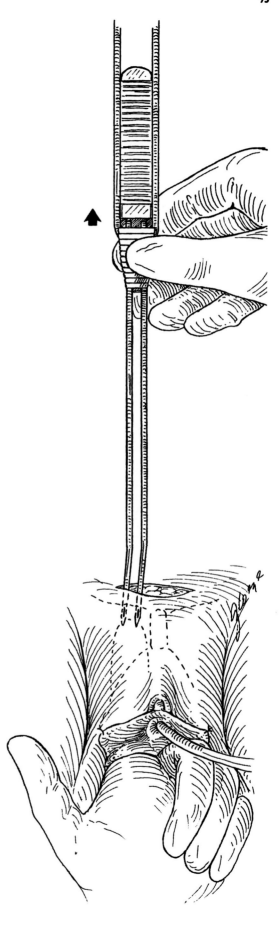

STEP 4:

Using a double-pronged needle and after preparation of the anterior vaginal wall as described earlier, we transfer the needle tips from the suprapubic to the vaginal area as in a bladder neck suspension. Four passes of the needle are required, and special attention must be paid to make this transfer as close as possible to the pubic bone (fixed area).

In the vaginal wall, the rectangular segment of fascia is fixed with absorbable sutures to the bladder neck area. Cystoscopy is performed, confirming proper coaptation and support of the urethra and bladder neck. The anterior vaginal wall is closed. In the suprapubic area the four sutures of Prolene are tied individually and without tension.

The procedure may be performed under local anesthesia in the office. One or two 7-ml tubes of Teflon paste are needed. The high density of the material makes injection difficult with the available syringes, so a special injector must be used to transmit the paste through the needle. For transurethral injection, a special pressure device and needle are required to fit a 21 to 23 cystoscopy sheath with 15- to 30-degree optics. For periurethral injection, a Lewy high-pressure syringe can be used.

The patient is in the lithotomy position. After preparation and draping, local anesthesia is given, using 2 per cent lidocaine jelly and 0.5 per cent lidocaine in the periurethral tissues.

Periurethral Injection (Fig. 5–3)

The Teflon paste is transferred to the high-pressure syringe connected to a 17-gauge needle. Under constant urethroscopy control, the needle is inserted periurethrally and in the submucosal tissues, avoiding intraluminal perforation. The needle is moved sideways in order to ascertain proper position in the proximal half of the urethra. The paste in injected (generally by an assistant) at three places: 2, 6, and 10 o'clock positions. Good elevation and apposition of the mucosa must be seen at the end of the procedure. One or two tubes may be injected.

Transurethral Injection

Using a special transurethral pressure syringe (Fig. 5–4), Teflon paste may be injected under direct vision underneath the urethral mucosa. The cystoscope is inserted into the bladder and the needle is advanced until only the tip is seen. The cystoscope is retracted into the mid and distal urethra, and under direct vision the tip of the needle is inserted underneath the urethral mucosa. With the help of an assistant the Teflon paste is deposited into the submucosal tissues, with constant observation for a possible leak of the paste and for a good bulking effect of the injection.

Postoperative Care

Postoperatively, a Foley catheter is left indwelling for 24 hours, and oral antibiotics are given. Pain is minimal with this procedure and responds to simple analgesics.

Complications

Recurrent urinary incontinence may occur because of poor tissue coaptation or leak of the paste into the urethral lumen. The inflammatory reaction and granuloma formation around the site of the Teflon paste takes a period of several weeks to subside. A second injection should not be attempted before 3 months.

Temporary urinary retention lasting 24 to 48 hours is expected after an injection. Permanent urinary retention is very rare, and self–intermittent catheterization may be initiated in selected cases. Infection of the injection site with formation of an abscess will lead to erosion and drainage of the collection into the urethral lumen. This ulceration will heal spontaneously and will not have any permanent adverse effect on the patient. Migration of Teflon particles has been reported experimentally to the local lymph nodes, lung, and brain, but no human case of death or carcinoma related to Teflon injections has been reported.

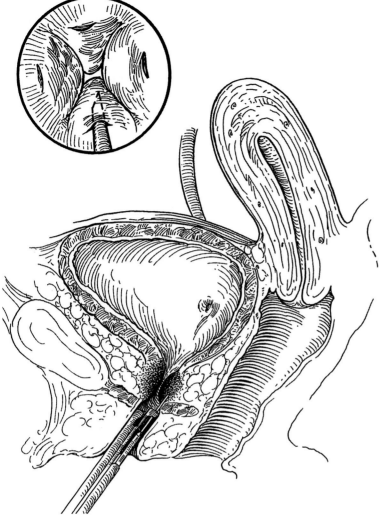

FIGURE 5—4. Teflon is injected periurethrally at the level of the proximal urethra and bladder neck.

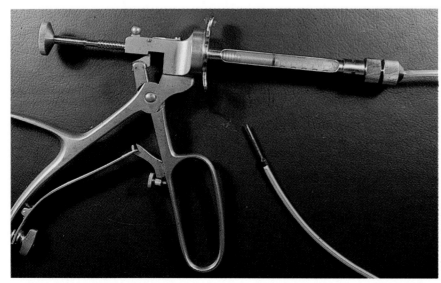

FIGURE 5—5. Special transurethral high-pressure injection system used with the Storz cystoscope.

Collagen Injections

Use of cross-linked collagen instead of Teflon has been studied experimentally and clinically. Good initial results have been reported. Collagen is easy to inject and does not require special equipment. Success has been reported in patients with urinary incontinence due to intrinsic sphincter damage, but use of collagen is not yet approved by the Food and Drug Administration.

TRANSURETHRAL OR PERIURETHRAL INJECTION OF AUTOLOGOUS FAT

Periurethral Injection of Autologous Fat

Indications

This a relatively new method of treatment by which fatty tissue is extracted from the lower abdomen by liposuction and injected trans- or periurethrally. The goal of the treatment is to provide coaptation of the sphincteric unit. Its main indication is in patients with urinary incontinence caused by intrinsic sphincteric dysfunction. The long-term effectiveness of fat injections is unknown at this time. The technique is simple, avoids the use of foreign material like Teflon or collagen, and may be repeated if required.

Diagnosis

The ideal candidates are patients with a clinical history of severe urinary incontinence who have good anatomic support. Cystoscopic examination confirms an open, fixed urethra; cystography confirms the presence of an open bladder neck. Video urodynamics confirm the presence of urinary loss without change in the true detrusor pressure, an open bladder neck, and a very low leak point pressure with stress.

Surgical Technique

The patient is placed in the lithotomy position. The suprapubic and vaginal areas are prepared. A sterile two-way receptacle (we use the Elik evacuator) is connected on one side to a large-bore hollow probe (7–10 mm) and on the other side to a high-pressure suction device. A small suprapubic stab wound is made, and the end of the probe is inserted. Using a back and forth maneuver, liposuction of 15 to 20 cc of fatty tissue is carried out, and the tissue is transferred to several 31 cc syringes for later use. The syringe is connected to a regular 18-gauge needle or angiocath. The periurethral injection of the fat is performed in at least three areas and under careful cystoscopic control to ensure proper location of the needle and good apposition of the mucosa. Alternatively, the injection may be performed transurethrally. Because of the low density of fat, fat injections do not require a high pressure injector.

FIGURE 5—6. Trocars used for liposuction of the lower abdominal wall.

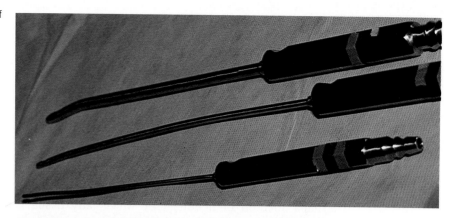

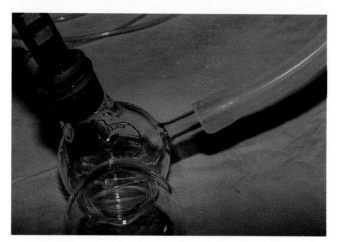

FIGURE 5—7. Elik evacuator modified so that one side is connected to the trocar and the other side to the high power suction unit.

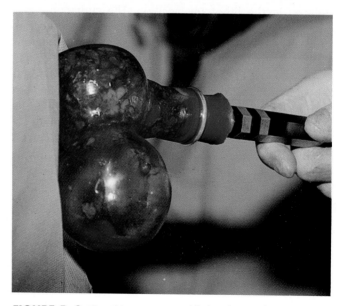

FIGURE 5—8. The Elik evacuator is filled with particles of fat with minimal serum or blood.

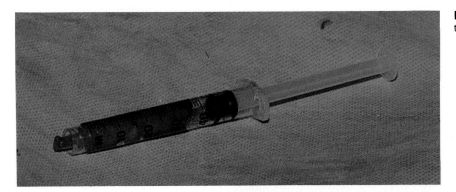

FIGURE 5–9. The fatty tissue is transferred to a 3-cc syringe and ready for injection.

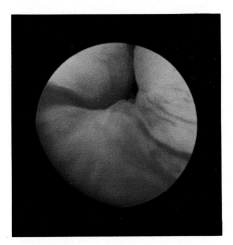

FIGURE 5–10. Urethroscopy after injection showing excellent coaptation of the urethral mucosa.

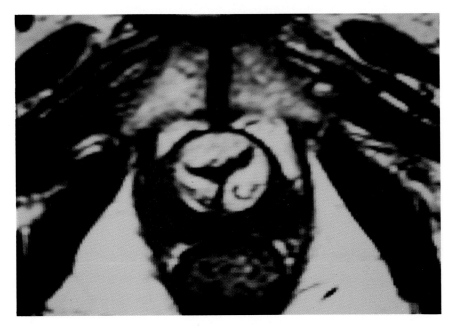

FIGURE 5–11. Magnetic imaging of the urethra of a patient after injection of fat. The urethral mucosa is displaced by the fatty tissue (in white).

VAGINAL PROLAPSE

The anatomic basis of vaginal prolapse was discussed in Chapter 1. The clinical presentation is in general that of a protruding vaginal mass, discomfort, pelvic pressure, and changes in bowel movement or urination. A careful diagnostic evaluation should include a medical, gynecologic, and urologic history. The vaginal, rectal, and bimanual examinations of the pelvis are helpful in determining the extent of the prolapse. Before anterocele or vaginal vault prolapse surgery is performed, objective assessment of the degree of bladder involvement is strongly recommended, because the supine physical examination can be misleading. It can be achieved by a standing cystogram that will provide information on the degree of urethral and bladder prolapse.

Surgical correction of severe and moderate bladder prolapse is described in Chapter 5. We will limit this discussion to the transvaginal surgical correction of rectocele, enterocele, and vaginal vault prolapse, and vaginal hysterectomy for severe uterine prolapse.

A. TRANSVAGINAL ENTEROCELE REPAIR

Indications

An enterocele is defined as a true hernia of bowel through the cul de sac, at the vaginal vault. When peritoneum and its contents herniate inferiorly into this space, an enterocele is formed. Although a congenital enterocele may be present in a woman without a previous history of vaginal surgery, most enteroceles are acquired as a result of the defect created at the vaginal apex between the widely separated uterosacral ligaments after hysterectomy. The most common manifestation of enterocele is a vaginal mass causing increasing pain and discomfort. Depending on the size of the mass, bowel incarceration may result.

The goal of surgery is to repair the hernia of the bowel that occurred at the Douglas pouch, plicate the cardinal and uterosacral ligaments, and provide support to the vaginal vault.

Diagnosis (Fig. 6–1)

On physical examination, the enterocele appears as a bulge high in the vagina, either posterior to the cervix, if it is present, or, as is most common

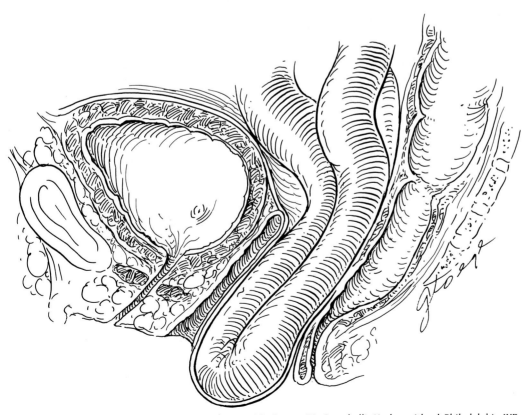

FIGURE 6–1. (From Walsh PC, Gittes RF, Perlmutter AD, Stamey TA: Campbell's Urology, 6th ed. Philadelphia, WB Saunders, 1992.)

following hysterectomy, at the apex of the vagina. Since an enterocele is frequently associated with a rectocele, the enterocele bulge may appear as a high continuation of the bulge in the posterior vaginal wall. The enterocele sac may contain bowel visible through the attenuated vaginal wall. With a finger in the rectum, the impulse of the enterocele hernia sac may be felt against the fingertip in the vagina during coughing (analogous to the impulse felt during examination for an inguinal hernia). When performing a bimanual rectal-vaginal examination, there is an increased thickness of the rectal-vaginal septum high in the vagina at the level of the enterocele. Physical examination in a standing position may help confirm the diagnosis in doubtful cases. Peritoneography with contrast dye also may be used. A voiding cystourethrogram (VCUG) is always performed to rule out the possibility that the bladder is part of the bulging mass. Magnetic resonance imaging (MRI) may be used in unusual cases.

Preoperative Considerations

Enterocele is commonly associated with other vaginal abnormalities (cystocele, rectocele, and so on), and the latter should be repaired simultaneously. Proper bowel preparation is required in case of accidental injury to the rectum or small bowel. After general or spinal anesthesia is induced, the patient is placed in the dorsal lithotomy position. The lower abdomen and vagina are prepped and draped in sterile fashion. The rectum is packed with Betadine-impregnated lubricated gauze and isolated from the surgical field.

Intraoperative Complications

Potential immediate complications include bleeding, ureteric injury, bladder or rectal perforation, and damage to the small bowel. Excessive bleeding may occur but is very rare.

Urinary tract bleeding (blood into the Foley catheter) requires cystoscopy to rule out bladder injury. Though the anterior retraction of the bladder should protect the ureters, ureteric injury may occur when the purse string sutures are placed. Intraoperative cystoscopy with intravenous injection of indigo carmine may be performed to assure the patency of the ureters. If the patient had adequate bowel preparation, any bowel injury can be repaired primarily. In case of stool contamination due to inadequate bowel preparation, a primary closure may be attempted with triple antibiotic coverage, but colostomy may be required in extensive injury.

Postoperative Care

The Foley catheter and vaginal packing are removed on the morning following surgery. Intravenous antibiotics are given for 24 hours, followed by oral antibiotics for several days.

SURGICAL TECHNIQUE

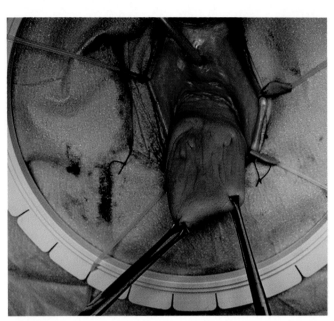

STEP 1:

A Scott retractor is positioned, and the labia are secured with special hooks. A Foley catheter is inserted to empty the bladder. When required, a weighted posterior retractor may be placed in the vagina and the labia retracted laterally with stay sutures.

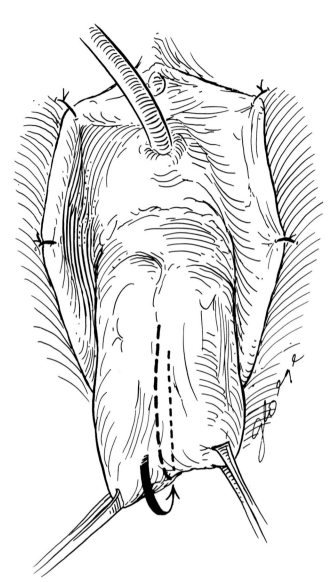

STEP 2:

The enterocele bulge is grasped with two Allis clamps, and 5 to 10 ml of normal saline is injected to facilitate dissection. A vertical incision is performed in the vaginal wall over the bulge. If the uterus has descended significantly, the enterocele repair can be performed only after its removal. (From Walsh PC, Gittes RF, Perlmutter AD, Stamey TA: Campbell's Urology, 6th ed. Philadelphia, WB Saunders, 1992.)

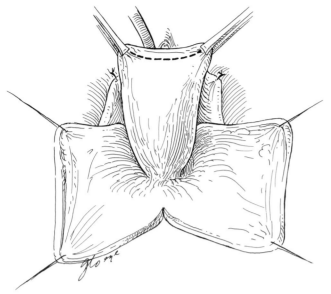

STEP 3:

After the vaginal wall is incised and dissected laterally, the peritoneal hernia sac is defined and separated from the vaginal wall, bladder, and rectum, using blunt and sharp dissection. The dotted line indicates the site where the sac will be opened.

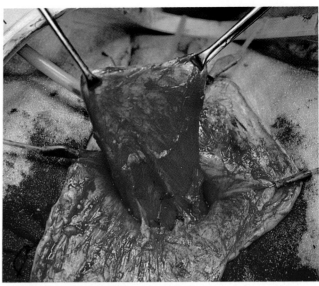

STEP 3 (continued):

The enterocele sac is isolated, and the hooks of the Scott retractor are reapplied at the vaginal wall to facilitate the exposure.

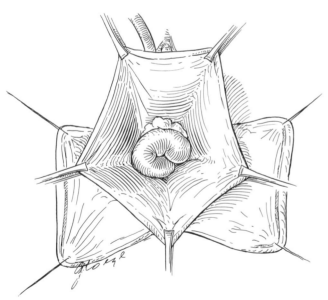

STEP 4:

The sac is opened, and any adhesions of the bowel are dissected free. (From Walsh PC, Gittes RF, Perlmutter AD, Stamey TA: Campbell's Urology, 6th ed. Philadelphia, WB Saunders, 1992.)

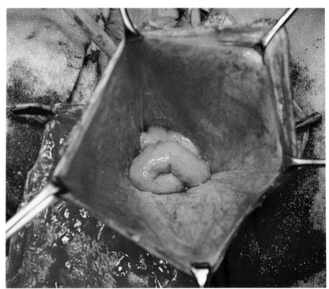

STEP 4 (continued):

The sac is exposed and dissected free of bladder and rectum up to the vaginal dome. A small laparotomy pad is inserted into the peritoneal cavity to protect the bowel during obliteration of the enterocele.

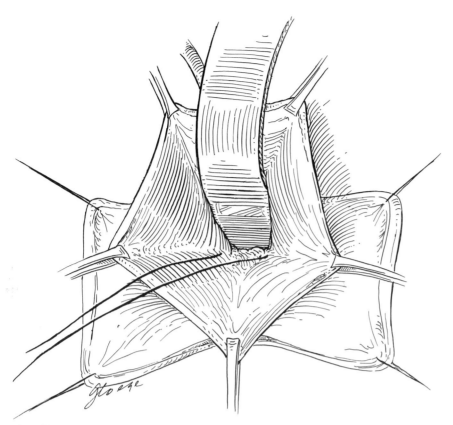

STEP 5:

Two purse string sutures Number 1 Vicryl are placed more proximally, incorporating the prerectal fascia posteriorly, the sacrouterine and cardinal complex laterally, and the bladder base anteriorly.

Another pair of sutures is applied to plicate the sacrouterine ligaments posteriorly. (From Walsh PC, Gittes RF, Perlmutter AD, Stamey TA: Campbell's Urology, 6th ed. Philadelphia, WB Saunders, 1992.)

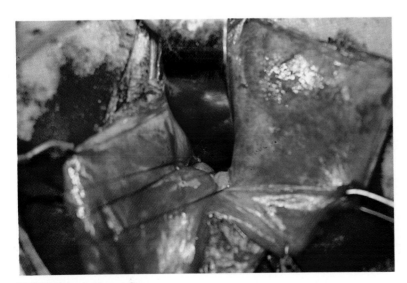

STEP 5 (continued):

A Deaver retractor applied anteriorly elevates the bladder base and trigone, protecting the ureters during application of the purse string sutures to the peritoneal sac.

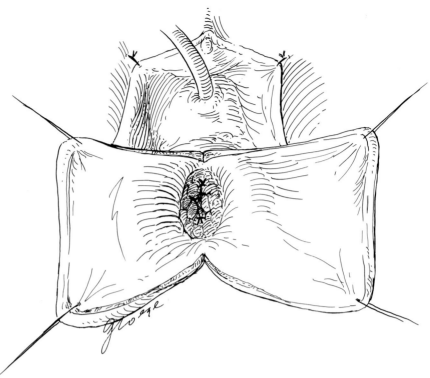

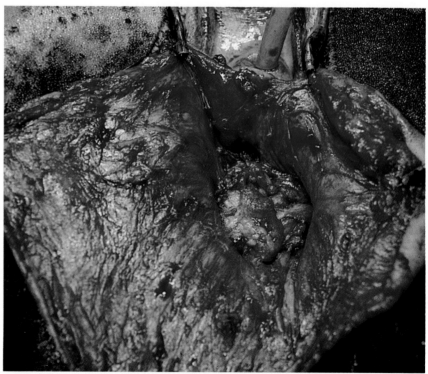

STEP 6:

After excision of the peritoneal sac, further approximation of the sacrouterine complex and prerectal fascia is accomplished with interrupted sutures of 2-0 Vicryl. (Drawing from Walsh PC, Gittes RF, Perlmutter AD, Stamey TA: Campbell's Urology, 6th ed. Philadelphia, WB Saunders, 1992.)

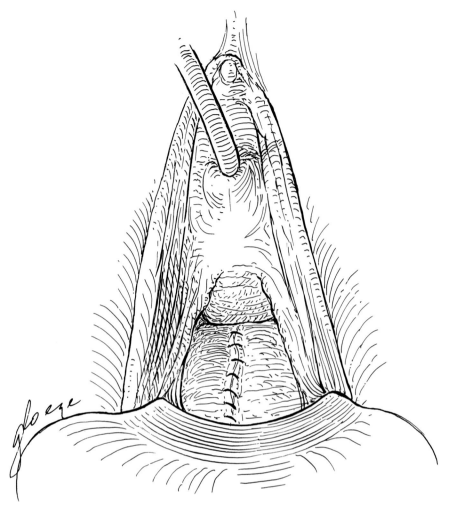

STEP 7:
The redundant vaginal wall is trimmed and closed with running 2-0 Vicryl sutures, incorporating the underlying fascia to avoid any dead space.

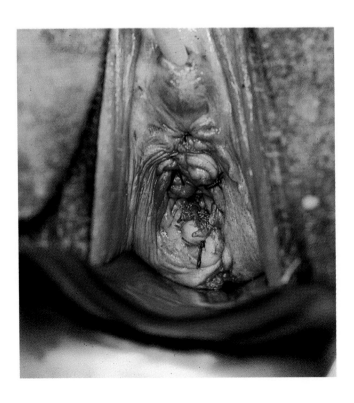

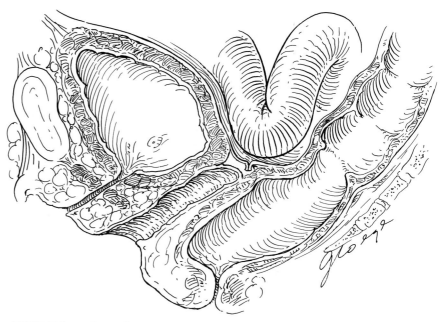

STEP 7 (continued):

A lateral view of the pelvis shows obliteration of the cul de sac by approximation of the vagina to the rectum. (From Walsh PC, Gittes RF, Perlmutter AD, Stamey TA: Campbell's Urology, 6th ed. Philadelphia, WB Saunders, 1992.)

Postoperative Complications

Late complications include vaginal shortening and recurrent enterocele. If the patient is sexually active and severe vaginal vault prolapse is present, we prefer to perform sacrospinalis fixation of the vagina with minimal excision of the vaginal wall. In sexually inactive patients, partial colpocleisis can be performed. Recurrent enterocele is very rare and should be repaired in a similar fashion or using a transabdominal approach.

B. POSTERIOR VAGINAL WALL REPAIR

Indications

Posterior repair is performed in conjunction with perineorrhaphy to correct a rectocele and to reconstruct a lax perineal body. A rectocele is a hernia that develops when the prerectal fascia and levator sling are insufficient to support the anterior rectal wall.

Perineal body laxity caused by attenuation of the perineal muscles usually accompanies a rectocele, and therefore reconstruction of the posterior fourchette is carried out at the same time. Surgery is performed not only when symptoms are present but also in patients with asymptomatic rectocele as part of other vaginal reconstructive procedures of the anterior vaginal wall (like bladder neck suspension or cystocele repair). Failing to do so may exacerbate posterior vaginal prolapse as well as diminish the chances for successful cure of urinary incontinence.

Diagnosis

Although rectocele is generally asymptomatic, the patient may complain of a bulging mass through the vagina, mostly with straining, that can be combined with difficulties in evacuation of stool. Some patients have to manually reduce the prolapsed posterior vaginal wall to obtain proper evacuation.

On pelvic examination the rectocele appears as a bulge in the posterior vaginal wall. The anterior rectal wall is palpated, and the extent of the rectal herniation into the posterior vagina is readily demonstrated. The degree of associated laxity and attenuation of the perineum, which results in a large, gaping introitus, should be assessed.

Occasionally there may be a coexistent enterocele that appears as a bulge higher in the posterior vaginal wall or at the vaginal apex. The preoperative appreciation of both these types of herniation is essential for proper surgical correction.

Preoperative Considerations

Forty-eight hours prior to surgery the patient is started on a clear liquid diet combined with laxatives. Upon admission, tap water enemas and intravenous antibiotics are administered.

Intraoperative Complications

Rectal injury is the major complication that can follow rectocele repair. This is prevented by careful development of the plane between the vaginal wall and the rectum. The rectal packing can assist in this dissection. Because of the preoperative rectal preparation and preoperative antibiotics, a rectal injury can be repaired primarily in multiple layers of absorbable sutures.

Excision of an excessive segment of posterior vaginal wall should be avoided because it may lead to vaginal stenosis and shortening.

Postoperative Care

The Foley catheter and vaginal packing are removed on the morning following surgery. The patient resumes a normal diet immediately after surgery. Intravenous antibiotics are given for 24 hours, followed by oral antibiotics for several days. Stool softeners are prescribed for a few days.

Postoperative Complications

Recurrent rectocele owing to poor tissue or closure under tension may require a secondary repair. Inadequate repair and approximation of the levator muscles will not correct the vaginal axis and may facilitate the recurrence of the rectocele or another vaginal prolapse.

SURGICAL TECHNIQUE

STEP 1:

The patient is placed in a dorsal lithotomy position. The lower abdomen and vagina are prepped and draped in a sterile fashion. The rectum is packed with Betadine-soaked gauze and isolated from the operative field with double draping. The labia are retracted laterally with stay sutures. A urethral Foley catheter is inserted and the bladder is drained. Upward traction of the anterior vaginal wall with a Deaver retractor and a ring retractor with hooks applied to the lateral vaginal wall provides good exposure.

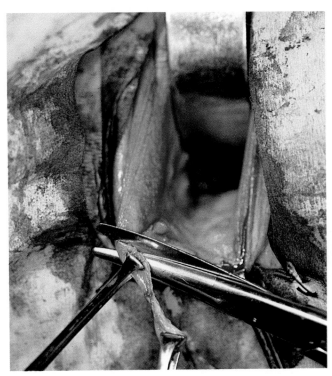

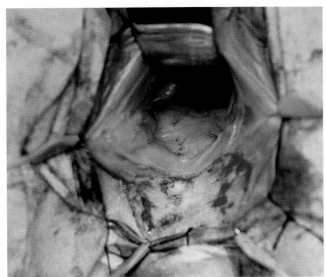

STEP 2:

Two Allis clamps are applied to the posterior margin of the introitus at approximately the 5 and 7 o'clock positions. These clamps are placed so that when they are brought together in the midline, the introitus readily admits two large fingers. A triangular flap of the mucocutaneous junction is then excised between these two clamps using curved Mayo scissors. Dissection is carried out laterally to expose the medial edge of the levators from the skin. The superficial perineal muscles are generally atrophied and not used in the perineal repair, but if present they are repaired in a separate subcutaneous layer. (Drawing from Walsh PC, Gittes RF, Perlmutter AD, Stamey TA: Campbell's Urology, 6th ed. Philadelphia, WB Saunders, 1992.)

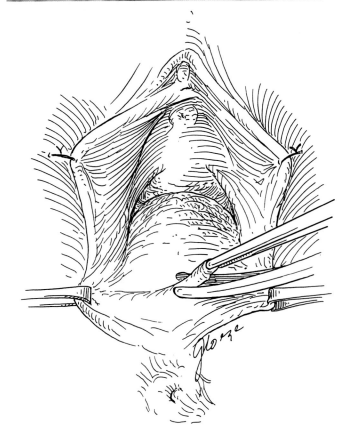

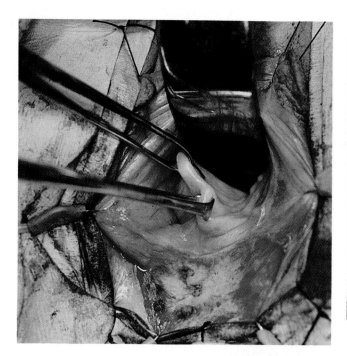
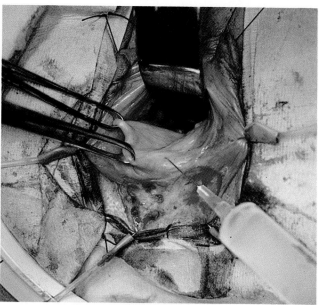

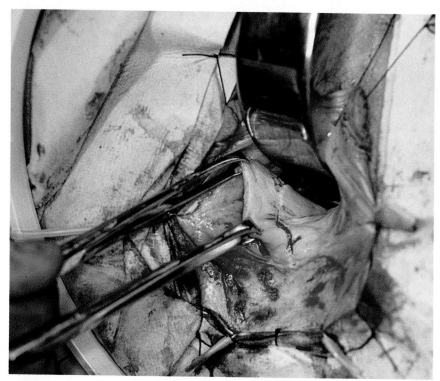

STEP 3:

Two Allis clamps are applied to the posterior vaginal wall overlying the rectocele, and the vaginal wall is infiltrated with 5 to 10 ml of normal saline to facilitate the dissection. While elevating the two Allis clamps, a triangular incision is made in the posterior vaginal wall, with the top of the triangle at the apex of the rectocele and its base along the previously made perineal incision.

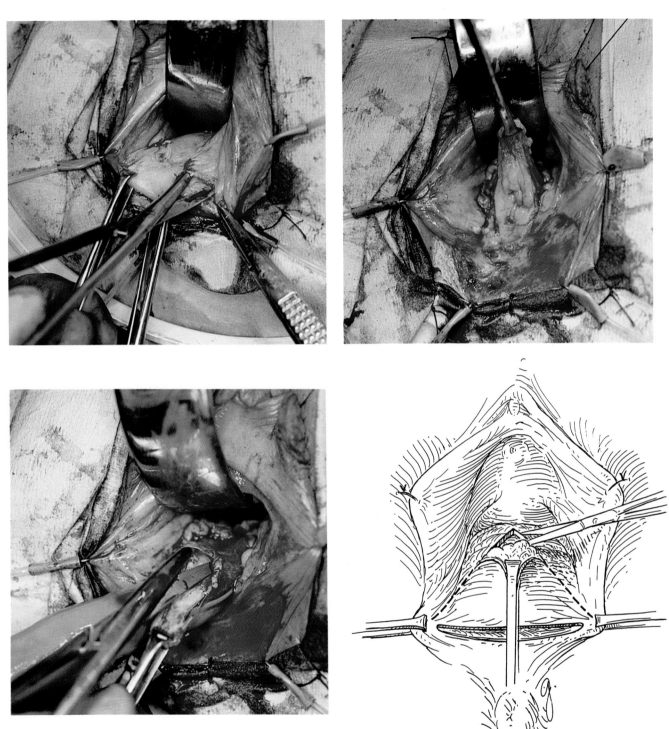

STEP 4:

With sharp dissection, a plane is developed between the herniated rectal wall and the vaginal epithelium, exposing the attenuated prerectal fascia. The dissection must stay as close to the vaginal epithelium as possible to avoid any injury to the rectal wall. Sharp dissection is continued laterally to expose the pararectal fascia. Palpation of the previously placed gauze in the rectum during the dissection facilitates identification of the rectum and helps avoid rectal injury. The isolated triangle of vaginal epithelium is excised. (Drawing from Walsh PC, Gittes RF, Perlmutter AD, Stamey TA: Campbell's Urology, 6th ed. Philadelphia, WB Saunders, 1992.)

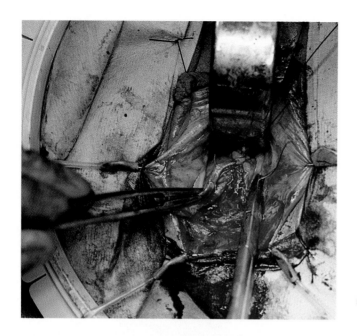

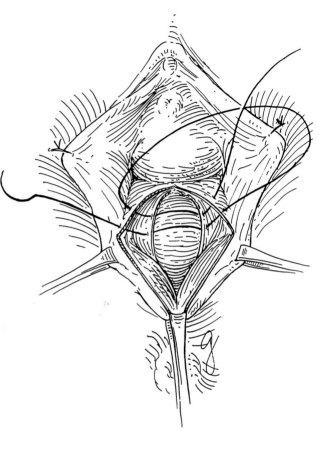

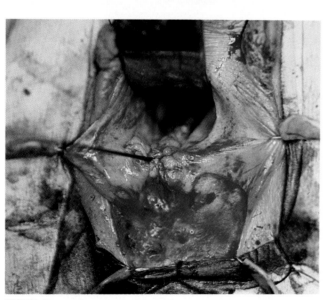

STEP 5:

Repair of the rectocele defect in the posterior vaginal wall is carried out. The rectum is protected by downward retraction of the bulging rectal wall with a narrow Deaver retractor over a folded gauze square. The rectocele repair is performed in a single layer, running locking number 2-0 polyglycolic acid suture, starting at the apex of the rectocele. The sutures incorporate the edge of the vaginal epithelium and a generous bite of the prerectal fascia, which is approximated in the midline over the rectocele. The levators are included in the distal one third of the closure.

The closure is carried down to the transverse perineal incision. The approximation of these layers should create a strong support and a smooth line of suture of the posterior vaginal wall. Upward retraction of the anterior vaginal wall with a proper retractor will help avoid narrowing of the vaginal wall during this part of the closure. (Drawing from Walsh PC, Gittes RF, Perlmutter AD, Stamey TA: Campbell's Urology, 6th ed. Philadelphia, WB Saunders, 1992.)

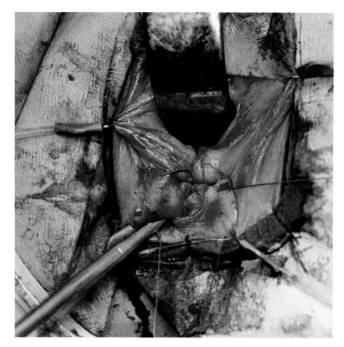

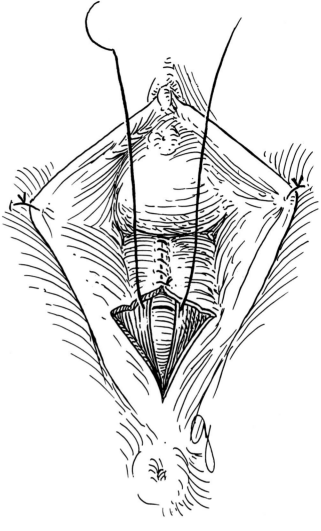

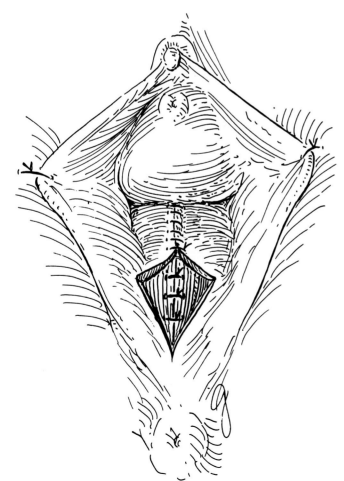

STEP 6:

The perineal laxity is corrected by using two or three Number 2-0 polyglycolic acid sutures in a vertical mattress fashion to reapproximate in the midline the weakened and separated pubococcygeus muscle. The superficial and deep transverse perineal muscles, and bulbocavernosus muscle if present, are approximated to recreate the perineal floor and central tendon.

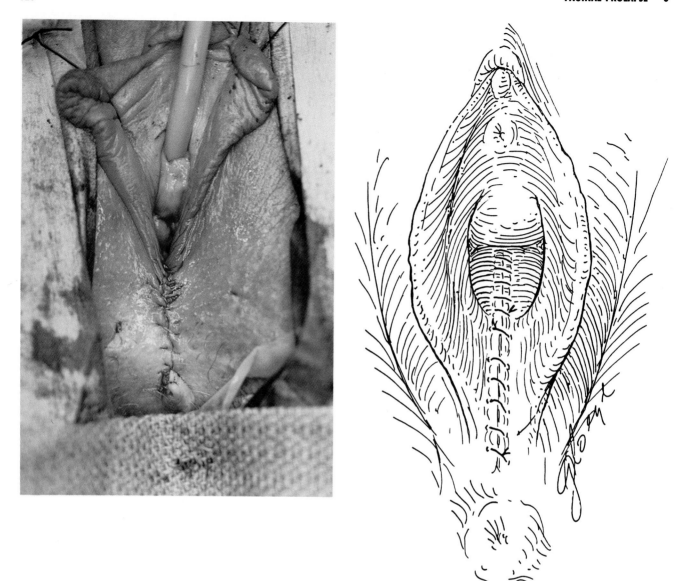

STEP 7:

The defect in the perineal skin is closed with a running Number 4-0 Vicryl suture. (Last drawing from Walsh PC, Gittes RF, Perlmutter AD, Stamey TA: Campbell's Urology, 6th ed. Philadelphia, WB Saunders, 1992.)

C. VAGINAL HYSTERECTOMY FOR SEVERE UTERINE PROLAPSE

Indications

Vaginal hysterectomy is generally necessary in cases of severe vaginal prolapse with concomitant uterine descent. Operations to provide support of the uterus are indicated in selected young patients. Uterine prolapse is rarely an isolated condition; associated pelvic floor relaxation and prolapse of the bladder and rectum are very common and should be repaired simultaneously. If severe (Grade IV) cystocele is present, we prefer to perform a vertical incision in the anterior vaginal wall, dissect the bladder free, reduce the cystocele, and then proceed with the hysterectomy. In cases of moderate cystocele, we perform the vaginal hysterectomy first, close the vaginal cuff, then perform a four corner bladder and bladder neck suspension. In this section we will describe vaginal hysterectomy for severe uterine prolapse as an independent procedure.

Contraindications

Vaginal hysterectomy is not routinely indicated in patients with good uterine support who are suffering from stress incontinence: hysterectomy has no impact on continence after surgery. Relative contraindications include uterine size out of proportion to vaginal accessibility, adnexal tumor, acute or subacute pelvic inflammation, endometriosis, and malignancy of ovaries or uterus.

Diagnosis

The diagnosis of uterine prolapse is easily made during a physical examination that reveals significant uterine descent. A clinical history of pelvic discomfort, vaginal mass, dyspareunia, or stress urinary incontinence associated with uterine prolapse is very common. Any history of vaginal bleeding must be fully evaluated to rule out uterine carcinoma. A bimanual pelvic examination will help grade the degree of uterine prolapse from minimal (to midvaginal area), moderate (midvagina to introitus), or severe (when the uterus is always outside the introitus). Any associated pelvic abnormality like cystocele, rectocele, enterocele, stress incontinence, or pelvic floor relaxation should be clearly defined because of the need of simultaneous repair. If required, imaging by ultrasound or computed tomography may help rule out other pelvic pathology.

Intraoperative Complications

Potential complications at the time of surgery include bleeding, which may be severe if the uterine artery or vein is lacerated prior to complete lateral exposure, ureteral injury, and bladder laceration.

Postoperative Care

Intravenous antibiotics are given for 24 hours. If no fever is present after 24 hours, an oral cephalosporin is given. The vaginal packing is removed the morning after surgery. Patients are discharged on the second day after surgery.

Postoperative Complications

Postoperative ureteral injury occurs with a frequency of less than 0.5 per cent, with the distal pelvic ureter immediately preceding its entrance into the bladder being the most commonly involved segment. Bladder fistula is seen less frequently and usually occurs either cranially along the bladder base or at the trigone.

Another potential complication is secondary enterocele due to laxity of the sacrouterine and cardinal complex. Vaginal stenosis and shortening may occur if the cul de sac is inappropriately closed.

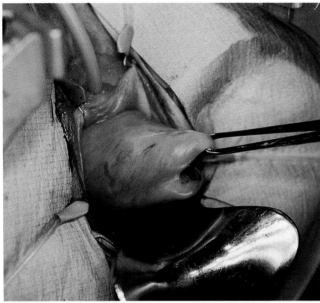

STEP 1:

The cervix is grasped with a tenaculum and brought outside the introitus. The exposure is facilitated by a ring retractor with multiple hooks.

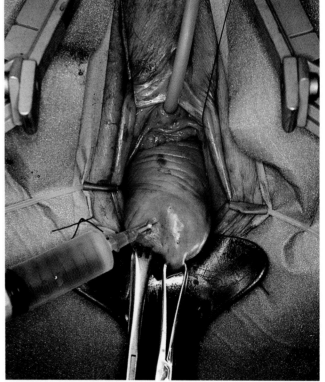

STEP 1 (*continued*):

Normal saline, without vasoconstrictors, is injected around the cervix. If suspension of the bladder neck or cystocele repair is to be carried out simultaneously, a suprapubic Foley catheter will be placed. A urethral catheter is also inserted. A weighted vaginal speculum with a glove at the end is inserted. A ring retractor with multiple hooks is used to retract the vaginal margins. The cervix is grasped with two single-toothed tenacula, and the mobility of the uterus is once more assessed.

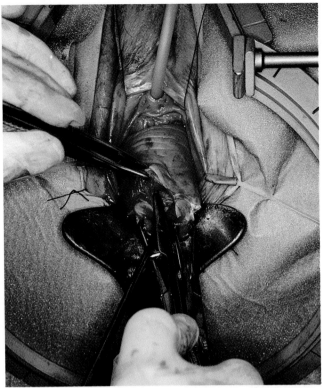

STEP 2:

A circular incision is made around the cervix. Blunt and sharp
dissection is carried out, using Metzenbaum scissors, in the
plane between the anterior cervix and the posterior bladder wall
and perivesical fascia.

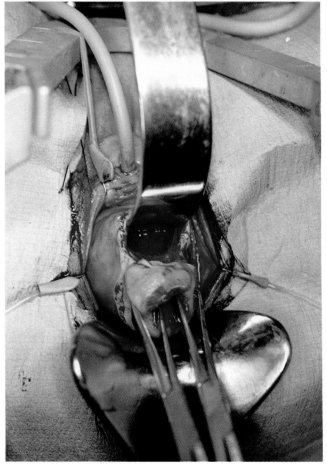

STEP 2 (continued):

A retractor is placed on the anterior vaginal wall to separate the
bladder from the cervix. With upward retraction, the pubocervical fascia and its anterior fusion to the cardinal ligaments are
now visualized. Dissection continues in an anterior direction
until the vesicouterine fold of peritoneum (anterior cul de sac) is
reached. Care is taken to avoid dissection laterally at this point.

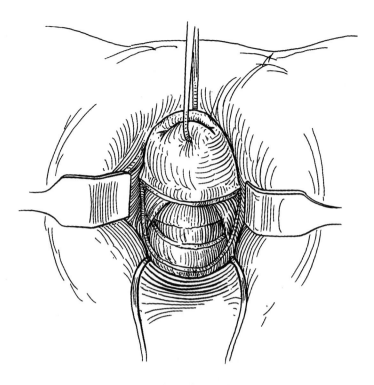

STEP 3:

With upward traction over the cervix, the dissection is carried out over the posterior cervical fascia.

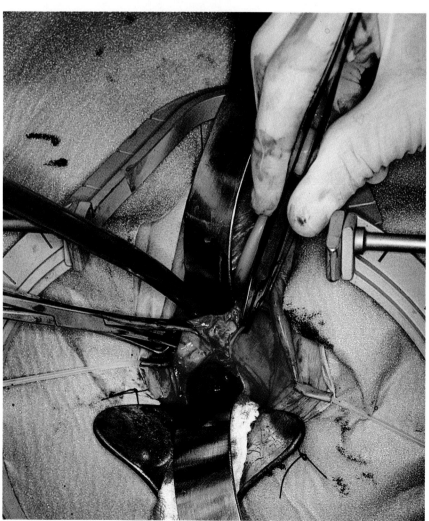

STEP 3 (*continued*):

Similar dissection is now carried out posteriorly, separating the posterior vaginal wall from the posterior fascia of the uterine cervix. After the rectum has been dissected away the posterior peritoneal fold (Douglas pouch) becomes visible. The posterior peritoneum is sharply open, flush to the uterus, and the angled retractor is placed in the open cul de sac.

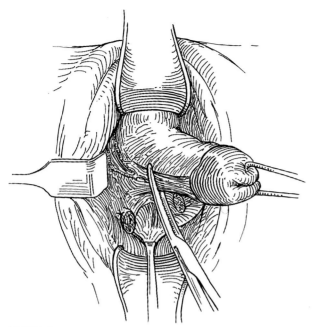

STEP 4:

The next step is to divide the cardinal and sacrouterine ligaments. These attachments are stretched by unilateral traction on the cervical tenaculum.

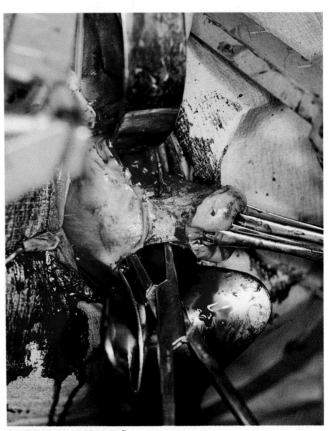

STEP 4 (*continued*):

The tip of a large right-angle clamp is introduced in the cul de sac at the level of the cervix. Pointing anteriorly, the attachment of the sacrouterine and cardinal ligaments is isolated as they attach to the cervix. One to two centimeters lateral from the cervix, the ligaments are individually clamped, divided, and ligated with a figure eight suture ligature. The suture ends are left long, clamped, and anchored lateral to one of the grooves of the ring retractor. The same maneuver is performed on both sides.

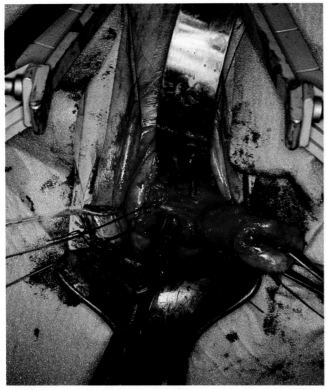

STEP 5:

The angled clamp isolates the uterine artery on the right. The cardinal and sacrouterine ligaments have been already ligated and incised, exposing the free length of the cervix.

With slight lateral traction of the cervix, the uterine artery and vein are identified and ligated individually on each side as they run lateral to the cervix. The suture ends are left long and anchored to one groove of the ring retractor.

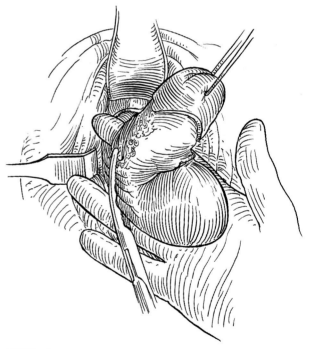

STEP 6:

The fundus of the uterus is everted and brought outside the introitus. With the anterior retractor elevating the bladder and mild posterior retraction of the uterus, the anterior peritoneal fold is visualized and entered. The thin, semilunar folds of peritoneum can now be visualized attaching to the uterine fundus. These folds are held with forceps, incised with scissors, and spread open. The anterior retractor is now introduced in the anterior peritoneal space. The uterus is now attached only by the broad ligaments on each side.

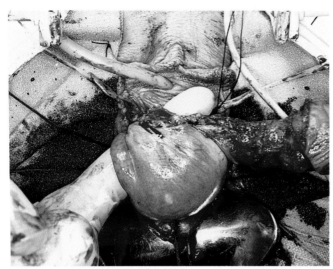

STEP 7:
The broad ligament on the right is exposed after the fundus of
the uterus has been everted.

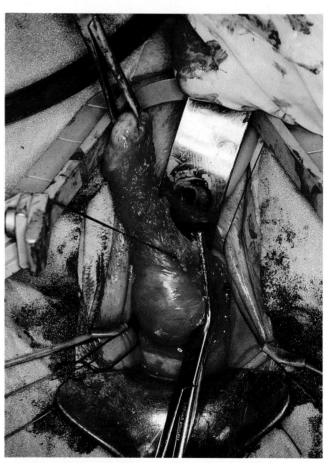

STEP 7 (*continued*):
A clamp is applied to the right broad ligament, close to the
uterine body.

  If the adnexa are to be left behind, their attachments must
now be ligated and severed at the uterine insertions. The side
chosen to divide first is best exposed by traction on the uterus
in the opposite direction. The utero-ovarian ligament, the fallopian tube, and the round ligament are visible in succession and
can be clamped, divided, and ligated with 2-0 Vicryl sutures in
one pedicle.

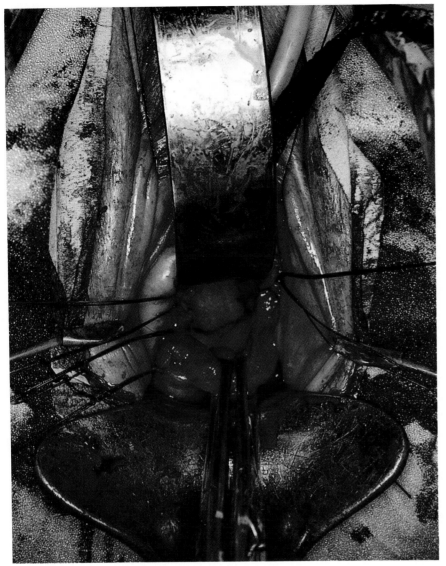

STEP 8:

After completion of the hysterectomy, three pedicles are observed on each side: the anterior includes the broad ligament, the middle represents the uterine artery, and the posterior includes the cardinal and sacrouterine ligaments.

The remaining parametrium, together with the tagged stumps of the cardinal and sacrouterine ligaments, is approximated—to the midline. The vaginal cuff is closed by a pair of purse string sutures (0-polyglycolic acid) that includes the prerectal fascia, the sacrouterine and cardinal complex, the broad ligaments, and the posterior bladder peritoneum. Plication sutures of the sacrouterine ligament are also applied. The beginning and end of these sutures are placed into the vaginal lumen so that during closure of the cuff, the vaginal wall is well supported. The vaginal mucosa is then closed with running 2-0 Vicryl sutures, and a vaginal packing with antibiotic cream is inserted.

D. SACROSPINOUS LIGAMENT FIXATION FOR VAGINAL VAULT PROLAPSE

Indications

In cases of massive vaginal vault prolapse, when limited cardinal and uterosacral ligament strength is demonstrated, the transvaginal sacrospinalis vaginal suspension is a suitable procedure for restoration of a functional vagina. The transvaginal approach to vaginal vault prolapse permits simultaneous correction of cystocele, enterocele, rectocele, perineal laxity, and uterine prolapse as part of the primary operative procedure.

Patients selected for this procedure must have proper bowel preparation and perioperative intravenous antibiotics. An unexpected rectal injury could be repaired primarily if the bowel was well prepared, whereas rectal injury with an unprepared bowel may require a diverting colostomy.

Diagnosis (Fig. 6–2)

The patient's symptoms are generally those of a vaginal mass protruding outside the introitus. On physical examination significant uterine prolapse may be found. In patients who have had a hysterectomy, a large enterocele is present with prolapse of the vaginal vault. Associated rectocele and cystocele are commonly found and should be treated at the same time.

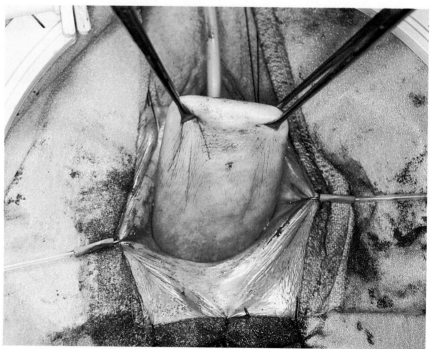

FIGURE 6–2. Intraoperative photograph of severe vaginal vault prolapse and enterocele.

Intraoperative Complications

A potential complication is bleeding, which can be significant if the pudendal vessels are injured; nerve damage to the pudendal or sciatic nerves may occur if the sutures are placed too laterally or too posteriorly. Another potential complication is rectal injury during the dissection or retraction of the pararectal space. This operation must be performed under full lower bowel preparation and parenteral antibiotics.

Postoperative Care

The vagina is packed with a vaginal packing coated with an antibiotic cream. The urethral and suprapubic catheters are connected to closed bag drainage. The suprapubic tube is secured in place with a 2-0 nylon suture.

The Foley catheter and vaginal packing are removed on the morning following surgery. Intravenous antibiotics are given for 24 hours, followed by oral antibiotics for several days.

Postoperative Complications

Some patients may complain of low back pain radiating from the back of the thigh following the procedure. This is a rare complaint that should respond to analgesics and time. Recurrent prolapse of the vaginal dome may occur because of laxity of the tissues. Another reason for failure is incomplete or poor anchoring of the vaginal dome into the sacrospinous ligament area. A transabdominal approach may be necessary in recurrent cases.

SURGICAL TECHNIQUE

STEP 1:

The patient is placed in a dorsal lithotomy position. The lower abdomen and vagina are prepped and draped in a sterile fashion. The rectum is packed with Betadine-impregnated lubricated gauze and then isolated from the operative field. The labia are retracted laterally with stay sutures. A suprapubic cystostomy tube is placed and a urethral catheter inserted. The bladder is emptied. A ring retractor is positioned and fixed with hooks.

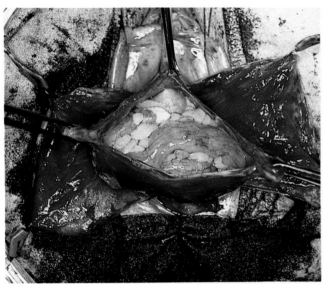

STEP 2:

After the enterocele sac has been opened and the bowel herniation reduced, the enterocele sac will be repaired. (See Section A on enterocele repair in this chapter.)

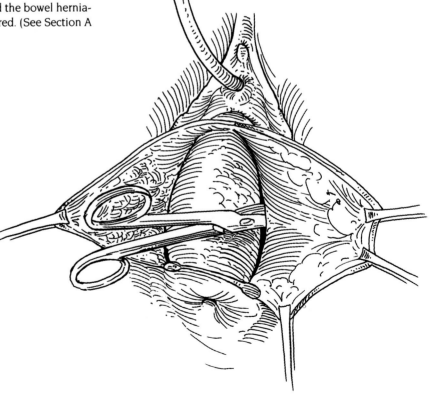

STEP 2 (continued):

A longitudinal incision is made in the posterior vaginal wall, exposing the prerectal fascia. Either the right or left rectal pillar, which separates the rectovaginal space from the pararectal space, is penetrated by blunt or sharp dissection. The pararectal space is beneath the peritoneum, above the levator floor. The opening in the rectal pillar is widened, exposing the superior surface of the pelvic diaphragm, including the coccygeus muscle, which contains the sacrospinal ligament.

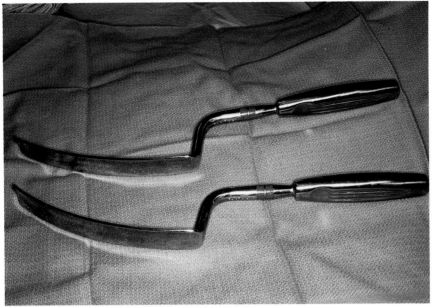

STEP 3:

Deep retractors, like the Breisky-Navratil, are required to retract the rectum medially
and expose the deeply located sacrosopinal ligament.

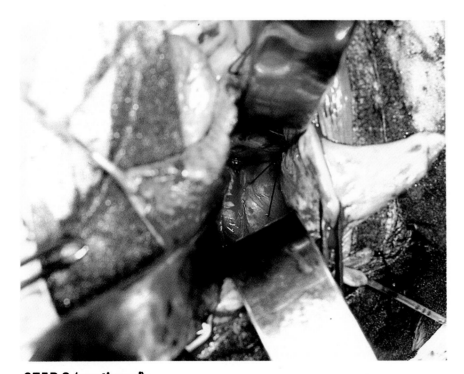

STEP 3 (*continued*):

A long retractor is inserted into the pararectal space, displacing the bladder and
peritoneum anteriorly. A second retractor displaces the rectum medially. Loose areo-
lar tissue is pushed to the side, and the pelvic surface of the coccygeus muscle–
sacrospinal ligament complex is identified running posterolaterally from the ischial
spine toward the sacrum.

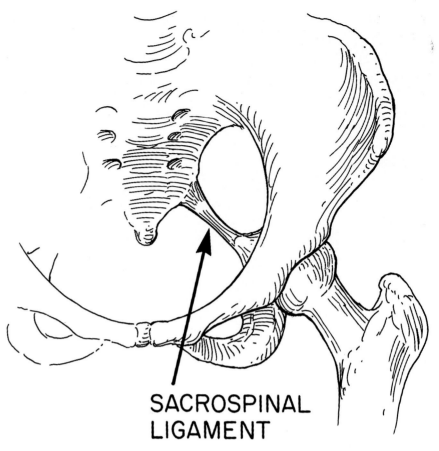

SACROSPINAL LIGAMENT

STEP 4:

The sacrospinal ligaments run between the ischial spine and the lateral side of the sacrum. Beneath the lateral insertion of the ligament the pudendal nerve, artery, and vein are found. Any anchoring suture to the ligament should be performed a few centimeters medial to the ischial spine to avoid trauma to these structures. Using a long needleholder with Number 1 absorbable sutures, two threads are passed through the substance of the coccygeus muscle and the sacrospinal ligament at the predetermined point, 1 cm apart. Gentle traction on the free ends of the suture will test the strength of the anchor.

STEP 5:

The two free ends of each suture are individually passed through the full thickness of the vaginal wall at the dome about 1 cm apart, with the threads emerging at the epithelial side. The two sutures are placed in healthy vaginal tissue that is not traversed by an incision or suture line, about 1 to 2 cm apart. The sutures are left untied but secured with a clamp, to be tied later after the hysterectomy or rectocele or enterocele repair has been completed.

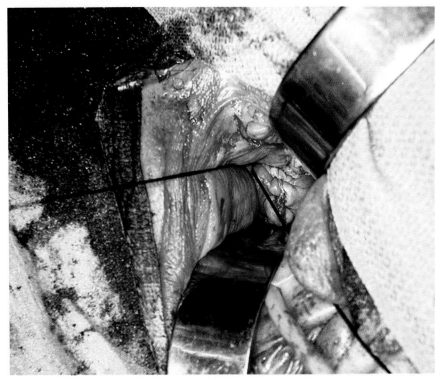

STEP 6:

After completion of the enterocele repair and closure of the vaginal wall, the two Number 1 absorbable sutures fix the vaginal wall to the left sacrospinal ligament.

The previously placed sutures in the sacrospinal ligament are tied individually, with the vaginal dome being directed under finger guidance to the uppermost position, where a square knot of the suspension sutures affixes it to the sacrospinal ligament on one side.

E. VAGINAL VAULT NEEDLE SUSPENSION FOR SEVERE PROLAPSE

Indications

Sacrospinalis fixation of the vaginal wall is a well established surgical procedure in the treatment of vaginal vault prolapse. However, the deep dissection required for proper exposure, together with the potential complications of nerve damage, bowel injury and bleeding, has restricted its use. Most surgeons elect to perform transabdominal fixation of the vaginal dome to the promontorium.

As an alternative to sacrospinalis fixation, we have developed a transvaginal operation using principles similar to those used in cystocele repair. The vaginal vault is anchored with nonabsorbable sutures. Using a double-pronged needle, the sutures are transferred from the vaginal to the suprapubic area, where the sutures will be tied, suspending the vaginal dome to the superior rami of the symphysis.

Indications for surgery and the diagnosis are similar to those of sacrospinalis fixation. We use this procedure exclusively in cases of vaginal vault prolapse with concomitant cystocele repair or bladder neck suspension surgery.

Complications

The potential complications of this procedure are the same as those of a cystocele repair (Chapter 5) or a vaginal hysterectomy (Chapter 6). The main advantage of the vault suspension is avoiding any perirectal dissection or placement of deep retractors with the potential of rectal injury. Also eliminated is the need for difficult and sometimes blind placement of sutures to the sacrospinalis ligament; thus we can avoid damage to the pudendal pedicle or the sciatic nerve.

SURGICAL TECHNIQUE

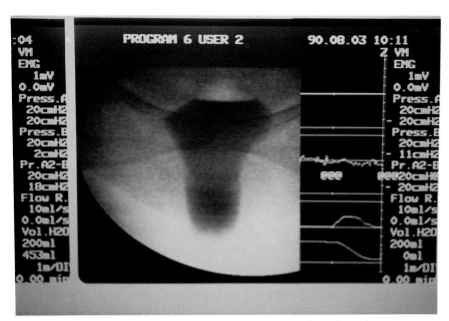

Video urodynamic study of a patient with severe vaginal vault prolapse (uterine prolapse) and a moderate cystocele.

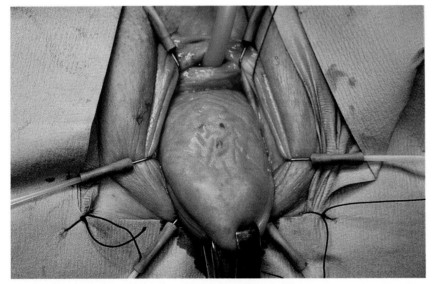

View of the anterior vaginal wall, showing the degree of uterine descent and associated cystocele.

If the cystocele is moderate or mild, two oblique incisions are made in the anterior vaginal wall; the periurethral fascia is dissected, the retropubic space is entered and another pair of suspending sutures will be applied to the vaginal wall at the level of the bladder neck (minus the epithelium) and the urethropelvic ligaments.

If the cystocele is severe (grade IV), a vertical incision is made, and the cystocele is reduced and repaired as described elsewhere. Another pair of prolene sutures will include the urethropelvic ligaments and the pubocervical fascia at the level of the bladder neck.

Four prolene sutures will support the anterior vaginal wall. An anterior pair supports the bladder neck and urethra, and a posterior pair will support the vaginal dome, including strong anchoring bites of the cardinal ligament and sacrouterine complex.

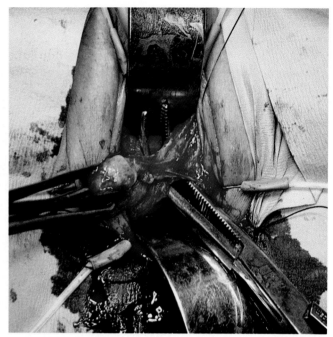

Vaginal hysterectomy is performed. The cardinal ligaments are isolated and will be tied individually.

A small suprapubic incision is made in the anterior vaginal wall. With a double-pronged needle and with the index finger in the retropubic space, the tip of the needle is transferred from the suprapubic to the vaginal area under the guidance of the finger. The four sutures are transferred individually. We must make sure that the passage of the ligature carrier is performed as close to the midline as possible and very close to the superior margin of the symphysis. This maneuver will obviate undue pain after surgery. Because of the design of the needle, a 1 cm bridge of anterior abdominal fascia is present between each suture. After injection of indigo carmine intravenously, cystoscopy is performed to ascertain that there is no bladder penetration, that the ureters are intact, and that elevation of the supporting sutures elevates the bladder base and bladder neck to the normal retropubic position.

The anterior vaginal wall is closed with a running suture of 2-0 absorbable material and the sutures of prolene are tied individually over the fascia without tension. The suprapubic wound is closed with intradermic sutures.

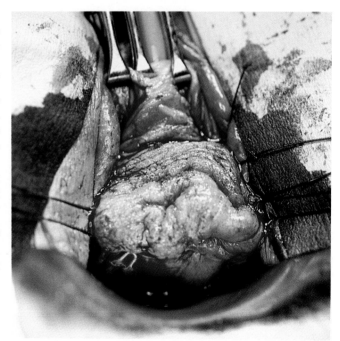

Four prolene sutures have been applied to the anterior vaginal wall. The proximal sutures include the vaginal wall, the cardinal ligament, and sacrouterine complex. The two distal sutures include the urethropelvic ligaments and the vaginal wall at the level of the bladder neck.

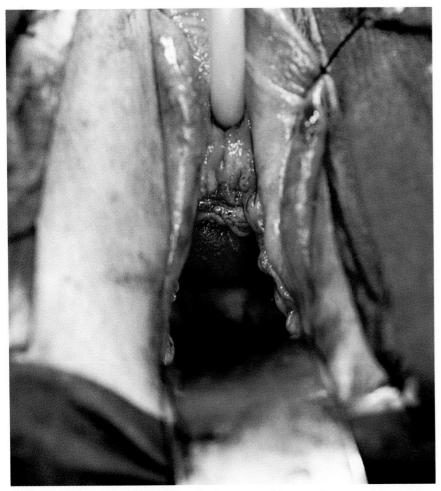

Elevation of the suspending sutures in the suprapubic area demonstrates excellent support of the vaginal dome and anterior wall.

VESICOVAGINAL

FISTULAS

The appearance of a urinary fistula to the vagina is one of the most devastating postoperative complications. The emotional distress of the patient and the surgeon is high because of the little hope that conservative therapy offers and the need in the majority of cases for a second operation to correct the problem. The long period of waiting for the final treatment while requiring use of multiple pads and the constant urinary leakage in spite of a Foley catheter add further stress to the patient. In developed countries the most common cause of vesicovaginal fistulas is gynecologic surgery, specifically hysterectomy. Other causes include urologic surgery or manipulation, trauma, gastrointestinal surgery, and radiation therapy for pelvic malignancies. Fistulas resulting from obstetric trauma are more common in developing nations.

Symptoms/Presentation

An unaccounted increase in vaginal drainage and the occurrence of bloody urine immediately after hysterectomy suggest fistula formation. Most vesicovaginal fistulas classically present as continuous day and night incontinence following a recent pelvic operation. However, a watery vaginal discharge accompanied by normal voiding may be the only sign of a small fistula.

Fistulas related to radiation therapy may develop up to 20 years after therapy, and recurrent tumor must be considered. Ureterovaginal fistulas may present as continuous leakage from the vagina with normal voiding, if only one ureter is injured.

Diagnosis

The clinical history and pelvic examination will aid in diagnosis. The bladder may be distended with methylene blue–dyed saline or indigo carmine–dyed saline and the site of leakage identified in the vagina. Cystoscopy (Fig. 7-1) and vaginoscopy may demonstrate the fistula's size, location, and relation to the ureteric orifices, as well as collateral fistulas. A biopsy of the site is mandatory in any patient with a history of pelvic neoplasm. Performing these studies under anesthesia may aid in diagnosis.

A second fistula, especially a ureterovaginal fistula in conjunction with a vesicovaginal fistula, is seen in up to 10 per cent of patients. Intravenous pyelogram may demonstrate partial or complete obstruction, suggesting a ureterovaginal fistula, but often the study can be completely normal. Retrograde pyelograms are more likely to demonstrate the exact location of a ureterovaginal fistula.

Cystogram or voiding cystourethrogram (VCUG) may demonstrate the extent of the fistula, the presence of vesicoureteral reflux, and associated urethral or vesical prolapse or stress incontinence, which may require simultaneous repair.

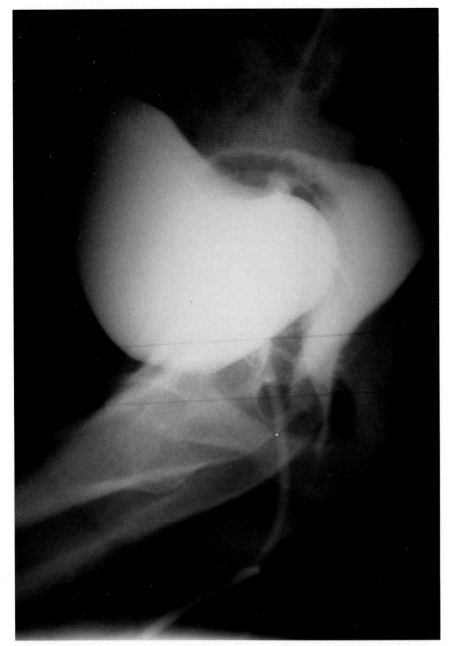

FIGURE 7–1. Cystogram of a patient suffering from a high vesicovaginal fistula after hysterectomy. Repair was by a transvaginal approach.

Principles of Surgical Repair

As soon as the diagnosis of fistula is made, a trial of conservative therapy should be started. These measures include adequate and undisturbed bladder drainage and antibiotics when indicated; in small fistulas fulguration of the area may be attempted. When conservative treatment has failed and the patient continues to leak most of her urine per vagina in spite of good bladder drainage, surgical correction of the fistula is necessary.

This condition requires sound surgical principles. The blood supply to the tissues must be adequate to support the area of repair. The tissues must be in optimal condition for repair—free of infection, excessive inflammation, and cancer. A layered closure should be utilized, with avoidance of overlapping suture lines. Suture material must be absorbable and cause little tissue reaction.

Continuous uninterrupted postoperative urinary drainage is critical to prevent extravasation and distention with breakdown of suture lines. Urethral and suprapubic catheter drainage are highly recommended.

In planning the treatment of vesicovaginal fistula, several important issues are considered: (1) the timing of surgery, (2) the surgical approach (abdominal, vaginal, or combined, (3) the use of estrogens or antibiotics, (4) whether or not to excise the fistulous tract, and (5) the use of adjuvant surgical measures to improve the fistula repair, such as Martius fibrofatty flaps from the labia.

Timing of Surgery

The timing of surgery remains a controversial issue. It is obvious that infection of the vaginal cuff or pelvic infection after abdominal hysterectomy requires prolonged antibiotic therapy before any attempted repair is made. The classic opinion regarding timing of the repair is to wait 3 to 6 months to allow the inflammatory reaction from surgical therapy to subside. This is particularly important if an abdominal approach is contemplated and the cause of the fistula was a complicated abdominal hysterectomy. Shortening the waiting period is very important to these "totally wet" patients. Early surgery would be of great psychologic benefit to the already distressed patients; however, one should not trade social convenience for a compromise on surgical success.

We favor early repair in the properly selected patient. We do not feel that a short waiting period of 2 to 3 weeks after the initial injury increases the risk, and the results are no different from those of the "long wait" approach, regardless of the route of repair. The patients are very satisfied by this early transvaginal repair because the emotional distress of long months of constant wetting is avoided.

Abdominal or Vaginal Approach

The best operation for repair of vesicovaginal fistula is the first operation. The selected route of repair depends mostly on the surgeon's training and experience. The best approach is probably the one that the surgeon feels most experienced in and comfortable with. We favor the vaginal approach because it avoids a laparotomy and the splitting of the bladder and provides a quicker recovery with less morbidity. We reserve the abdominal approach for rare cases when intra-abdominal pathology requires simultaneous care. The most common case is radiation cystitis and fistula, with a small, contracted bladder capacity requiring cystoplasty and fistula repair. Radiation fistula per se does not preclude the vaginal approach if the bladder capacity is appropriate.

Use of Estrogens and Antibiotics

The improved turgor and vascular supply of the vaginal wall after estrogen replacement in the postmenopausal or posthysterectomy patient may aid in healing of the vagina, and therefore estrogen therapy is strongly recommended.

Broad-spectrum antibiotics are required in any fistula repair, particularly if an early approach is used. Generally we like to use a combination of an aminoglycoside and a cephalosporin, starting 24 hours prior to operation. Because the vaginal area is usually contaminated and infected from the constant urinary drainage, we use an iodine solution to scrub with and for douching the vaginal area the night before and the day of operation.

Excision of the Fistulous Tract

The classic approach to the repair of vesicovaginal or any fistula includes wide excision of the fistulous tract to freshen the margins and provide a better repair.

In a series of 65 cases of early transvaginal repair of vesicovaginal fistula, we did not excise the fistulous tract, without apparent adverse effects. In our view, not excising the fistulous tract has many advantages. During repair, a small fistula stays small if not excised, but as soon as a fistulous tract is excised, a small opening becomes very large. Bleeding of the freshly excised margins may require coagulation of the edges, which compromises the closure. The fistulous tract provides a ring of protection against postsurgical bladder spasms that, if severe, may compromise the healing. When the fistulous tract is removed, this protecting ring is lost, and the fresh repair may be at higher risk if severe bladder spasms occur after operation. The greatest advantage in not excising the fistulous tract occurs when the fistula is very close to the ureteric orifices. In this situation, excision of the fistula will necessitate open surgery and reimplantation of the ureters; if the fistula is not excised, the ureter can be catheterized with a stent, and, under direct vision of the ureteric catheter, a safe transvaginal closure of the fistula can be performed, avoiding ureteric reimplantation.

Adjuvant Measures

In the majority of cases, uncomplicated vesicovaginal fistula requires only multilayer tension-free repair of the fistula. But when complicating factors like prior radiation, prior failed operation, or poor quality of tissues is present, adjuvant measures are required.

When the repair is done by an abdominal approach, omentum is commonly used. It is an excellent source of reinforcement and protection of a tenuous closure. Some surgeons use the omentum routinely when obtainable. In selected cases we have interposed the pericolonic or mesenteric fat.

Our technique of transvaginal repair of vesicovaginal fistula will be described later in detail, but in short includes no excision of the fistulous tract; multilayer, tension-free closure of the fistula; and the advancement of a vaginal flap, covering the area of the repair with healthy tissue. However, very often it is desirable or necessary to reinforce a routine closure. Several measures are available in this case: (1) use of fibrofatty tissue from the labia (Martius flap), (2) use of rotation flaps of the entire labia and/or gluteal skin, (3) use of myocutaneous gracilis muscle flaps, and (4) more recently we have used peritoneal flaps in the repair of high fistulas. This technique will be described later.

Use of Single J Stents

In selected cases, it is desirable to improve urinary drainage during the repair of a difficult fistula, such as one occurring after radiation therapy. In addition to placement of suprapubic and urethral catheters, bilateral single J ureteral stents can be inserted. For the first few days after surgery the bladder will be free of urine, permitting prolonged dryness of the repair site.

VAGINAL REPAIR OF SIMPLE/UNCOMPLICATED VESICOVAGINAL FISTULAS

The transvaginal approach for simple vesicovaginal fistulas offers several advantages: excellent exposure; no opening of the bladder or abdomen, resulting in reduced postoperative discomfort; minimal dissection resulting in minimal blood loss; interposition of viable tissue if needed; multilayer closure; possible correction of associated stress urinary incontinence; and shorter hospital stay.

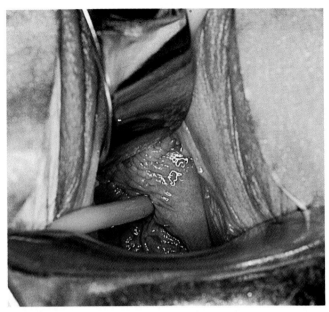

STEP 1:

After insertion of the suprapubic and urethral catheters, the fistulous tract is dilated and a third Foley catheter is inserted into it. This catheter will provide traction and improve exposure.

The patient is placed in the exaggerated lithotomy position. In a narrowed vaginal vault, increased exposure can be obtained by posterolateral relaxing incisions prior to insertion of the posterior weighted vaginal retractor. If the fistula is close to the ureteral orifices, cystoscopy and ureteral catheterization should be performed. A urethral catheter and a suprapubic catheter are placed by means of a Lowsley retractor. If required, the fistulous tract is dilated to 12 French, and a small 8 to 10 Foley catheter is inserted into the fistula. This catheter will provide excellent retraction and exposure at the time of initial preparation of the vaginal flaps.

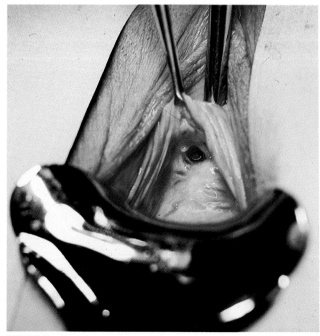

STEP 2:

Vaginal view of a recurrent vesicovaginal fistula after failed repair.

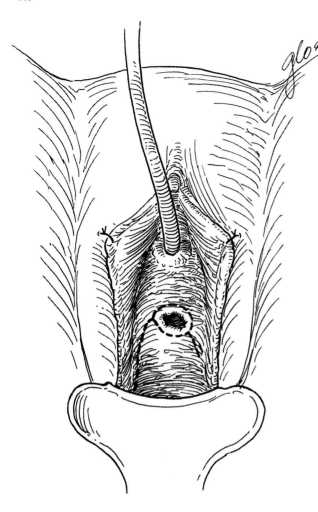

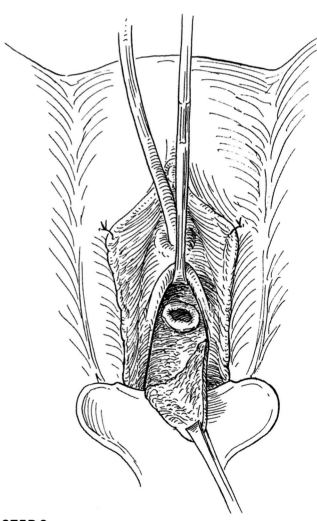

STEP 2 (*continued*):

Saline is injected into the anterior vaginal wall around the fistulous tract. An inverted **J** incision is made in the anterior vaginal wall. The long end of the incision extends toward the apex of the vagina. The convex portion of the incision circumscribes the fistulous tract. This asymmetric incision allows for the later advancement and rotation of the posterior flap over the fistula repair.

STEP 3:

Diagram showing the dissection of two flaps on the anterior and posterior side of the fistula. The ring of vaginal wall around the fistula is left intact.

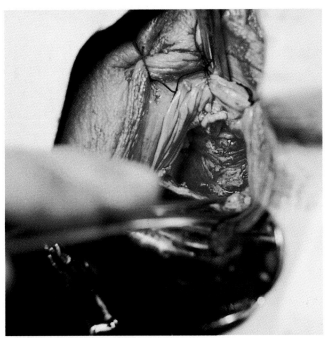

STEP 3 (continued):
Two flaps are created on the anterior and posterior sides of the fistula. Creation of the flaps is begun in healthy tissue away from the fistulous tract. This maneuver aids in the dissection of proper tissue planes, avoiding bladder perforation or expanding the fistulous tract.

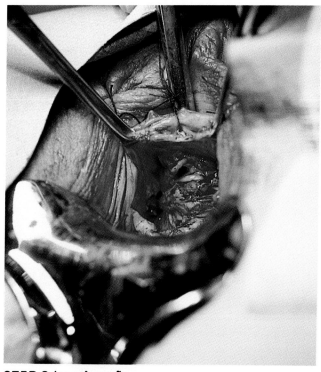

STEP 3 (continued):
The scarred margin of the fistula is left in place, and no attempt is made to dissect the thin layer of vaginal wall overlying the fistula. The dissection of the flaps is extended at least 2 to 4 cm from the fistulous tract, exposing the perivesical fascia.

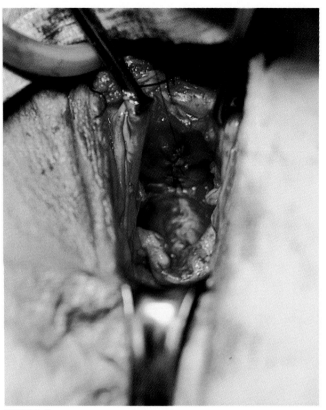

STEP 4:

Interrupted sutures 2-0 absorbable sutures (Vicryl or Dexon) are used to close the first layer of the repair. Included in this suture line is partial thickness of the bladder and the vaginal wall, which has remained connected to the fistulous tract. A strong bite of tissue 2 to 3 mm from the margin of the fistula is obtained. After application of the sutures, the intrafistula catheter is removed and the sutures are tied, closing the fistulous tract. A second layer of interrupted absorbable sutures is used to invert the prior layer. These sutures include the perivesical fascia and deep musculature of the bladder. The sutures should be applied at least 1 cm from the prior line of suture and tied free of tension. The first layer of the repair remains invaginated and covered by the second layer of sutures. At this time the bladder is filled with indigo carmine diluted in saline, testing the integrity of the repair.

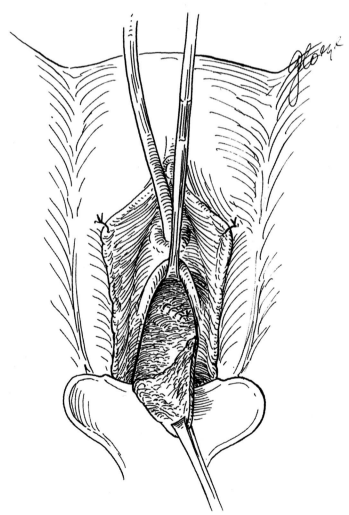

STEP 4 (*continued*):

Diagram showing the completed closure of the fistula, with the anterior and posterior flaps still intact. The entire fistulous tract should be covered entirely by the second layer of perivesical fascia.

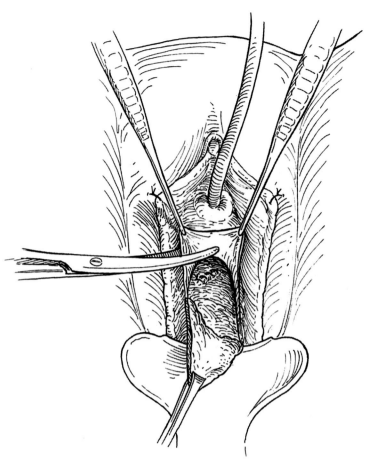

STEP 5:

The previously raised anterior flap is now resected.

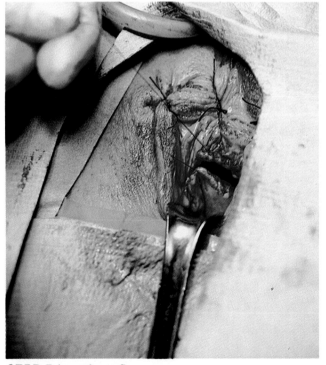

STEP 5 (*continued*):

The posterior (proximal) flap is rotated and extended beyond the closure of the fistula in order to cover the fistulous tract with fresh vaginal tissue and to avoid adjacent and overlapping suture lines.

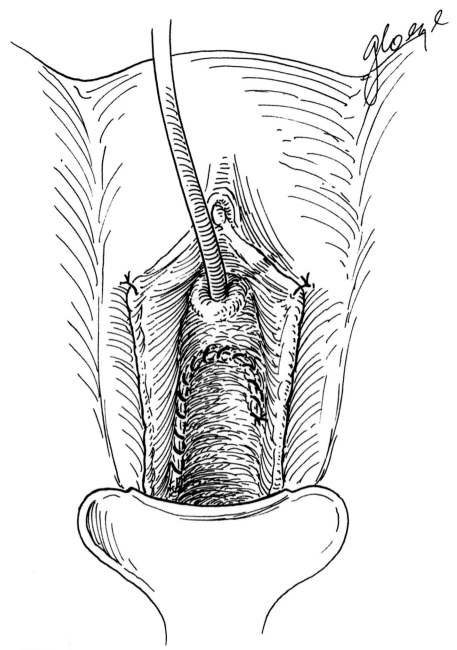

STEP 5 (*continued*):

A running suture of absorbable 2-0 material is used to complete this layer. The vaginal wall is advanced at least 3 cm beyond the fistula closure.

Intraoperative Complications

Bleeding can be a problem during the dissection of the vaginal flaps and should be controlled with fine, absorbable sutures. Although apical fistulas generally do not require ureteric catheterization, this maneuver is recommended for fistulas close to the trigonal area because of the higher risk of ureteric injury. If there is doubt, cystoscopy after injection of indigo carmine and ureteric catheterization should be performed to assure the integrity of the ureters. The strength of the first and second lines of closure is crucial for a successful outcome.

Postoperative Care

A dressing soaked in Betadine or triple sulfa is inserted in the vagina. The suprapubic and urethral catheters are connected to a leg bag.

The patient receives antibiotics until the Foley catheter is removed, and anticholinergics are prescribed to avoid bladder spasms. The patient is discharged from the hospital 2 days after surgery with instructions to avoid strenuous exercise but no other restrictions. The most important aspect of postoperative care is uninterrupted catheter drainage. The urethral catheter is removed on day 10 to 14 after operation, and a suprapubic cystogram is performed. If the outpatient cystogram documents vesical integrity, the suprapubic catheter is removed. Patients should abstain from sexual intercourse for 3 months.

Postoperative Complications

Immediate complications, like vaginal infection, bladder spasms, or vaginal bleeding, should be treated aggressively to avoid fistula recurrence. Perioperative antibiotics are important to avoid vaginal wall infection and should be continued as required. Bladder spasms may lead to breakage of the repair; they should be treated with cholinolytic agents and, if required, local anesthetics. Secondary vaginal bleeding should be treated with bed rest and vaginal packing if necessary. Vaginal stenosis and shortening may result from unnecessary excessive resection of the vaginal wall and may require secondary vaginoplasty. Unrecognized ureteric injury (leak or, more commonly, obstruction) may require percutaneous nephrostomy and a cooling off period. Endoscopy procedures, like retrograde catheterization or transurethral ureteroscopy, should be avoided in the immediate postoperative period; antegrade procedures are recommended.

The most important complication is recurrence of the fistula. With adherence to the basic principles of wide mobilization and tension-free closure, with multiple noncrossing layers, the repair will succeed in more than 95 per cent of cases. If it does recur, after a proper waiting period, the fistula can be repaired again through the vagina, but in this case a flap of fibrofatty labial tissue or peritoneum should be used.

SURGICAL REPAIR OF COMPLEX/RECURRENT VESICOVAGINAL FISTULAS

Most of the uncomplicated vesicovaginal fistulas do not require more than the simple technique just described. However, in cases of recurrent fistula, radiation or ischemic injury, poor quality of tissue owing to lack of estrogens, severe atrophy, and doubtful closure of the fistulous tract, we can use an array of procedures to enhance the quality of the repair.

Fibrofatty Labial Flap (Martius Flap)

This procedure allows for the advancement of a well-vascularized fatty tissue flap to the area of the surgical repair in recurrent procedures, in radiation fistulas (Fig. 7–2) or when in a simple repair the closure is not entirely satisfactory and tension free.

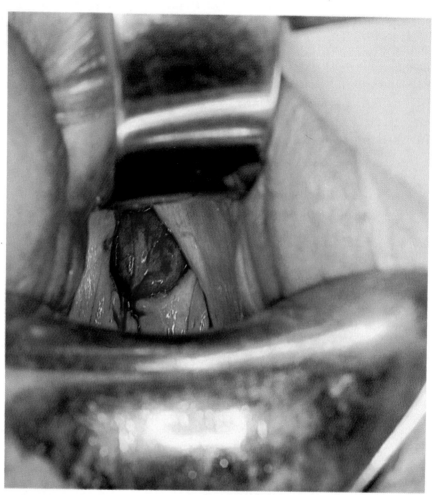

FIGURE 7–2. Large vesicovaginal fistula 10 years after radiation therapy for carcinoma of the cervix.

Peritoneal Flaps

The Martius technique is an excellent source of well-vascularized tissue, and its use is highly recommended in selected cases. One problem with the Martius flap is the atrophy of the labial tissue often found in postmenopausal patients. The tissue in these cases is very thin and poorly vascularized. Another problem of the Martius flap is the difficulty in reaching the vaginal apex in some cases of high fistula repair (the most common repair nowadays). To circumvent this problem, in the last 3 years we have initiated the use of peritoneal flaps as a means of providing an extra layer of cover to the fistula repair.

After the initial incisions are made, the posterior vaginal flap is dissected further posteriorly toward the peritoneal reflexion. The closed peritoneum is freed from its adhesion to the posterior bladder wall and advanced forward.

Rotational Labial Flaps

The entire labia majora (including skin and underlying fibrofatty tissue) can be used to cover a significant and difficult vaginal fistula. After completion of the fistula closure, attention is paid to the area of the labia majora. A longitudinal incision is made along the vaginal canal from the area of the repair toward the superior margin of the labia majora. A U incision is made in continuity to the prior incision around the labia, with its base at the posterior introital area. The medial and lateral sides of the U are 1 to 2 cm from the labia. Dissection is carried out deep into the adductor fascia and the inferior margin of the vagina. The flap will be reflected from the deep fasciae covering the pubic bone and will include, as a unit, the skin of the labia and the fatty tissue underneath. The whole flap is swung laterally to cover the area of the repair. The vaginal wall will be anastomosed with absorbable sutures to the edges of this rotational flap.

This technique is very useful in repairing a vesicovaginal fistula in cases of severe atrophic changes or small vagina. It provides a means of covering the fistula defect with fresh vascularized tissues and enlarging the vaginal canal at the same time. A possible contraindication of this procedure is the patient's concern about the external appearance of the vaginal introitus after surgery.

SURGICAL TECHNIQUE

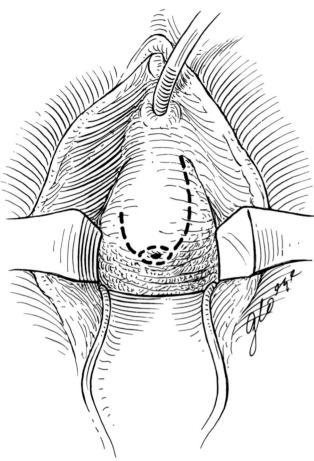

STEP 1:

Because of the high position of the fistula and local changes in the tissues, the inverted **J** incision has been modified. The incision circumscribes the fistula as a **J** incision.

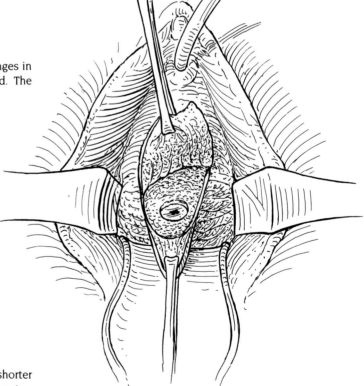

STEP 2:

A large anterior flap based toward the introitus and a shorter posterior flap are dissected free, isolating the fistulous tract.

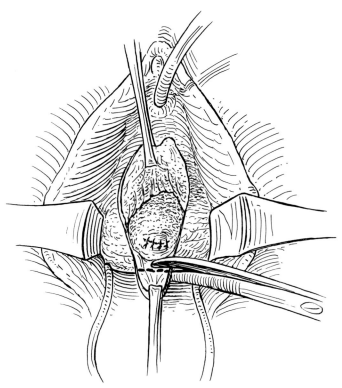

STEP 3:

The posterior vaginal flap is excised and the fistulous tract is closed in two layers as described earlier.

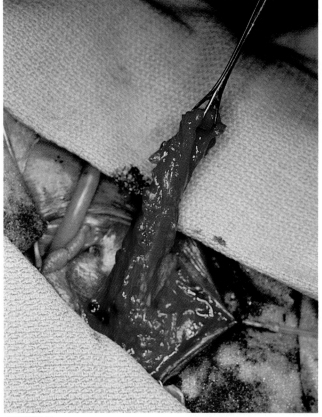

STEP 4:

A vertical incision is made over the labia majoris, and the subcutaneous tissues are dissected laterally. The fibrofatty pad of tissue extends from the anterior surface of the pubic bone to the base of the labia majoris, where it receives its main vascular supply. A small Penrose drain is used to isolate the entire thickness of the flap. The dissection is continued anterior and posterior. The anterior segment is clamped and transected anterior to the pubic symphysis. The free segment of the flap is now dissected from the underlying structures, obtaining a long and broad flap of fibrofatty tissue based posteriorly.

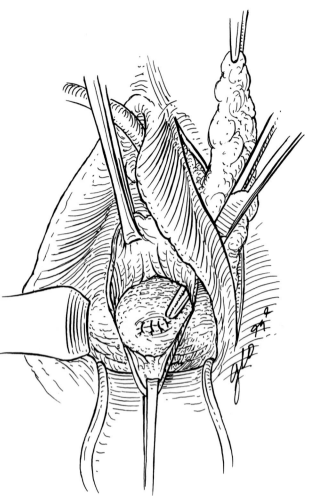

STEP 5:

Attention is now paid to the vaginal wall. Dissection is carried out between the vaginal wall and perivaginal tissues, creating a long tunnel from the labia majoris to the area of the fistula.

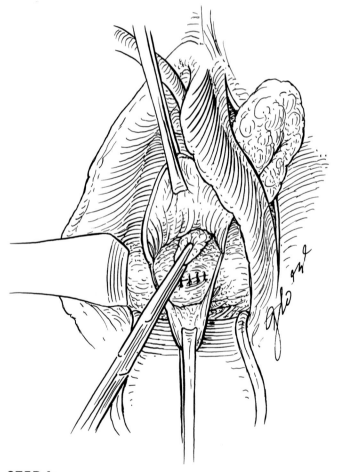

STEP 6:

The end of a hemostat clamp is transferred underneath the vaginal tunnel toward the labia. The end of the fibrofatty pad is transferred from the labial to the vaginal area. Tension should be avoided. Interrupted sutures are used to secure the fibrofatty tissue to the perivesical fascia, making sure to overlap the area of the repair.

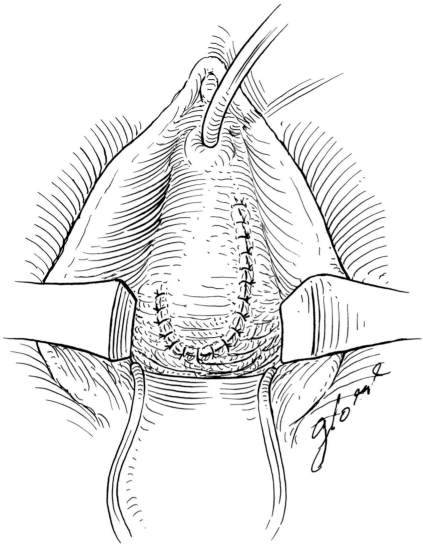

STEP 7:

The vaginal flap is advanced to cover the area of repaired fistula and fibrofatty graft.
After good hemostasis, the labial incision is closed with intradermic sutures, and a
small drain is left in place.

SURGICAL TECHNIQUE

Peritoneal Flap Technique

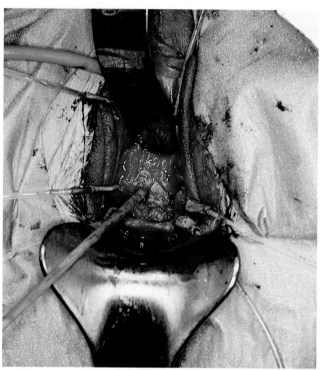

STEP 1:

High vesicovaginal fistula. After dissection of the flaps and perivesical fascia, traction on the intrafistula Foley catheter provides excellent exposure to the vaginal dome. The fistula will be closed in two layers.

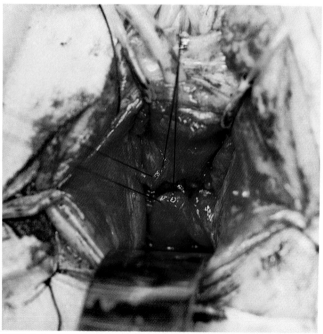

STEP 2:

The peritoneal flap, including preperitoneal fat, is advanced to cover the fistula repair. Interrupted sutures are used to anchor the peritoneum to the perivesical fascia, overlapping the fistulous tract repair. The last layer will be the advancement of the vaginal wall flap to cover the entire area.

Rotational Flaps of Gluteal Skin

The skin of the gluteal area can be used to cover a vaginal defect or fistula repair when no other tissue is available. After completion of the first two layers of fistula repair, a longitudinal incision is made in the vaginal wall toward the midportion of the labia majora. The labia are divided in two and separated with self-retaining retractors. An extended semicircular skin incision is made in the gluteal skin in continuity with the labial incision. After proper dissection and undermining of the skin, a flap is rotated and advanced into the vaginal canal. The area of the fistula is covered with the skin, and the edges of the vaginal incision are sutured to the edges of the flap. If desired, a second stage can be performed to incise the base of the skin flap and restore the labial anatomy to normal.

This technique is very useful in radiation fistula and in patients with a very short or unavailable vaginal canal.

Myocutaneous or Gracilis Muscle Flap

By this technique a bulky, well-vascularized flap of skin and underlying gracilis muscle is brought to the vaginal area. It is used in difficult cases of vesicovaginal fistula repair, in particular when the vaginal canal is very atrophic or absent owing to radiation therapy (Fig. 7–3). The gracilis flaps will

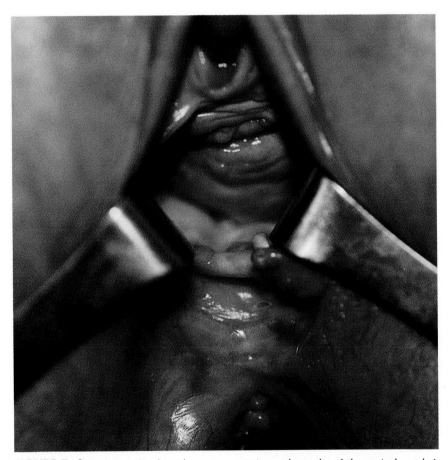

FIGURE 7–3. Radiation fistula with severe narrowing and atrophy of the vaginal canal. A myocutaneous flap will be used to cover the fistula repair and provide vaginal depth.

allow coverage of the fistula defect and reconstruction of a functional vagina. Bilateral flaps are often used.

Use of a viable gracilis muscle flap may enable the repair of a complex fistula. A long skin incision extends over the course of the muscle from the medial condyle of the femur to the inferior border of the symphysis pubis. Lying between the adductor longus laterally and the adductor magnus posteromedially, the tendinous part of the muscle is identified, divided, and held with stay sutures. During muscle dissection, it is important to preserve the blood and nerve supply entering the muscle along its lateral border. After adequate mobilization, the gracilis muscle is tunneled through the upper thigh and labia and into the vagina, where it is fixed with 2-0 Dexon or Vicryl sutures around the fistula.

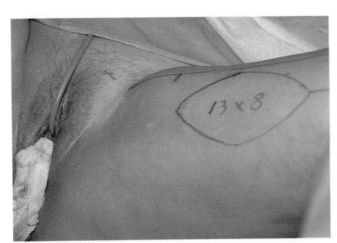

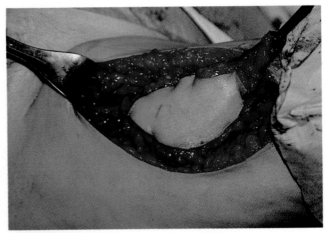

STEP 1:
A tennis racquet type of incision is made in the inner part of the thigh.

STEP 2:
Dissection is carried out to the subcutaneous tissues. The gracilis muscle is detached in its most distal part.

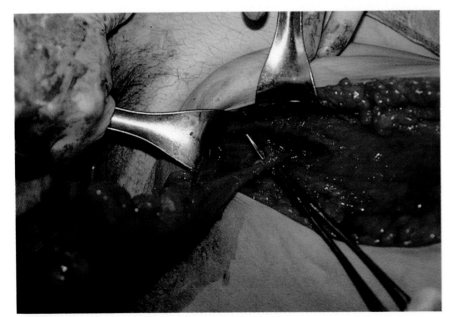

STEP 3:
After isolation of the skin and gracilis muscle, a pedicle is raised based on the proximal circulation of the gracilis muscle.

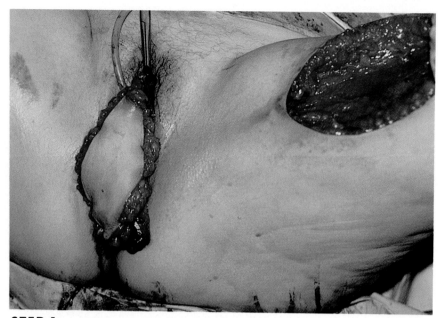

STEP 4:

A channel is made underneath the skin, and the flap is brought to the vaginal area.

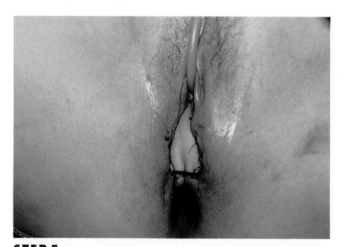

STEP 5:

The skin and muscular flap provide an excellent cover of the fistulous tract and can be used to reconstruct the vaginal canal.

Radiation Fistulas

Radiation vesicovaginal fistulas occur with an incidence of 1 to 5 per cent following radiation therapy of pelvic malignancy, in particular neoplasia of the uterus and cervix. Because of radiation-induced obliterative endarteritis, the area around the defect is poorly vascularized, thereby reducing the chances of spontaneous as well as surgical healing. The time delay between radiation therapy and fistula formation is variable but may be 15 to 20 years after the therapy was completed.

Preoperatively, the edges of the fistula and the surrounding tissue must be examined and a biopsy performed to rule out residual or recurrent cancer. Prior to operation, pelvic and upper tract imaging (intravenous pyelogram, pelvic computed tomography, or ultrasound) is strongly recommended to rule out pelvic mass or ureteric obstruction.

Time-honored principles, such as lack of tension, separated suture lines, and preservation of blood supply are not always sufficient to obtain a successful closure. Interposition of viable tissue may help in revascularizing the ischemic fistula region and provide a successful vaginal repair. The use of tissues in the immediate vicinity, such as peritoneal flap, bulbocavernosus muscle Martius flap, or gluteal or labial flaps, is highly recommended. In extensive cases, the likelihood of the tissues' exposure to some radiation renders them less than ideal for this purpose. Instead, a myocutaneous flap or the gracilis muscle should be brought from one or both sides.

The approach depends on the exact site of the fistula, the involvement of the ureteric orifices, the presence of collateral fistulas, the extent of the radiation field, the number of previous attempts at surgical repair, the sexual activity of the patient, and the experience of the surgeon.

In the presence of a small, contracted bladder capacity due to radiation cystitis, an enlargement cystoplasty is required. In this case we use an augmenting segment of small or large bowel to cover the area of the repair. In spite of radiation injury to the vagina, we prefer an initial vaginal repair for radiation fistula, except when an enlargement cystoplasty is required. The advantages of the vaginal approach include multilayer closure, advancement of vaginal flap, interposition of labial fibrofatty tissue, use of gracilis muscle flap or Martius flap, avoidance of bowel manipulation in a previously irradiated field, less blood loss, and decreased postoperative discomfort.

EXCISION OF
URETHRAL
DIVERTICULA

INDICATIONS

Urethral diverticula result in most cases from obstruction and inflammation of the periurethral glands. In rare cases they are congenital or traumatic following urethroscopy, urethrotomy, or an open surgical procedure. They are usually posterior and located in the mid and distal third of the urethra. They may be single or multiple, and the urethral communication may be wide or very narrow. Rarely urethral diverticula will occur in the anterior urethra or its proximal third. Distal urethral diverticula may originate from an obstructed Skene gland draining into the urethral meatus.

Surgical therapy is indicated in patients with significant symptoms related to the presence of the diverticulum. Symptoms include recurrent urinary tract infections, severe pain, dyspareunia, frequency, urgency and postvoid dribbling. It is not uncommon to have stress urinary incontinence and urethral hypermobility in conjunction with urethral diverticula.

Surgical options include (1) transurethral incision of the diverticular communication, transforming a narrow-mouthed into a wide-mouthed diverticulum, (2) marsupialization of the diverticular sac into the vagina by incision of the urethrovaginal septum, and (3) excision of the diverticulum. We will discuss only our technique of surgical excision of a large urethral diverticulum.

DIAGNOSIS

On physical examination, the urethra is found to be tender. Manual compression may lead to the expression of purulent material from the external meatus. The presence of urethral hypermobility and stress incontinence should be documented prior to surgery. The preoperative diagnosis of anatomic stress incontinence may warrant a combined operation to correct the diverticulum and the stress incontinence.

Urethroscopy should be performed using a zero-degree lens and a sheath with a very short beak, allowing the entire urethra to be distended for adequate visualization. Constant water flow and bladder neck occlusion at urethroscopy enhance the yield of the test. At endoscopy, the urethra is compressed, and any active drainage of pus from the mouth of the diverticulum is observed.

The postvoid film of an intravenous pyelogram will often reveal a collection of contrast in the subvesical area. The voiding cystogram in the oblique position is the most reliable diagnostic tool. This study will best define the location, size, and number of diverticula. In doubtful cases, positive pressure urethrography with a double balloon catheter can be used. In difficult cases, magnetic resonance imaging (MRI) or ultrasound of the urethra is a helpful tool to assess the extension and location of the diverticula.

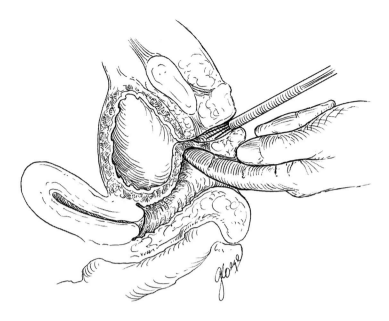

FIGURE 8–1. Diagram of urethroscopy with a 0-degree lens, showing the occlusion of the bladder neck when constant perfusion of fluid distends the urethra.

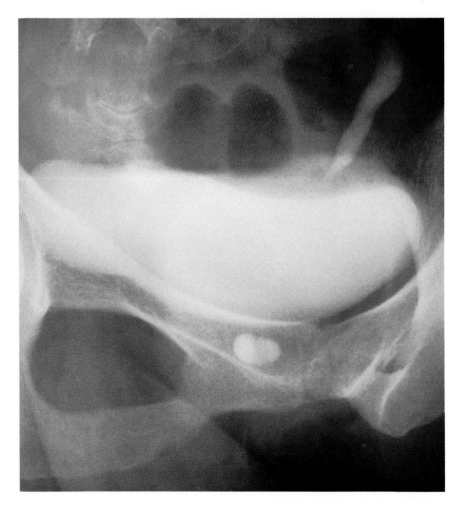

FIGURE 8–2. Postvoid film after intravenous pyelogram in a patient suffering from recurrent urinary tract infection. A diverticulum is seen in the midurethral area.

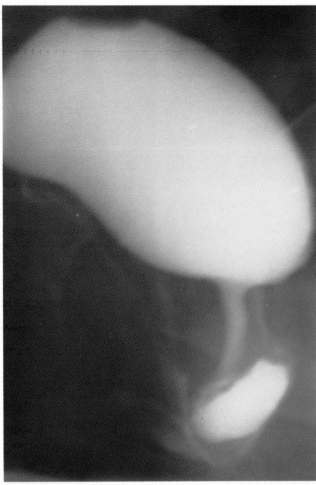

FIGURE 8—3. Voiding cystogram in a patient with recurrent urinary infection and pain during intercourse. A distal diverticulum is present.

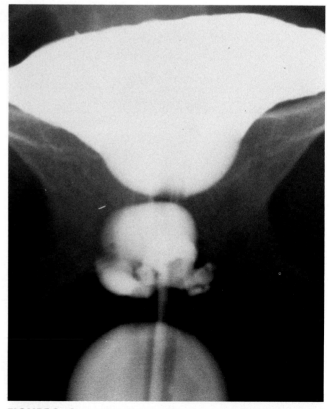

FIGURE 8—4. Double-balloon urethrogram in a patient with terminal dribbling and urinary tract infection. A large midurethral diverticulum is well seen.

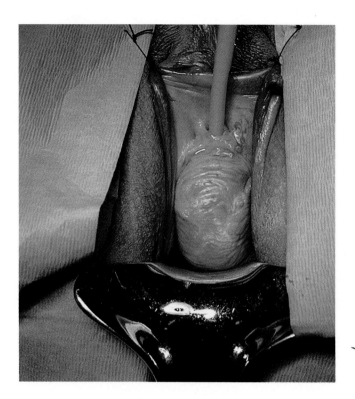

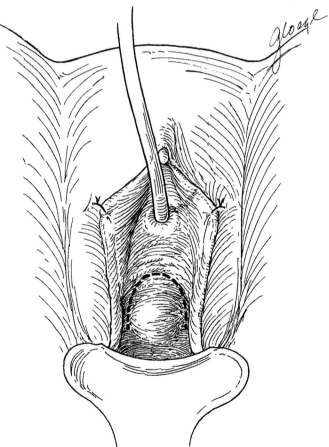

STEP 1:

After insertion of a posterior weighted retractor and urethral and suprapubic catheters (using a Lowsley retractor), an inverted U incision is made, with the apex just proximal to the urethral meatus.

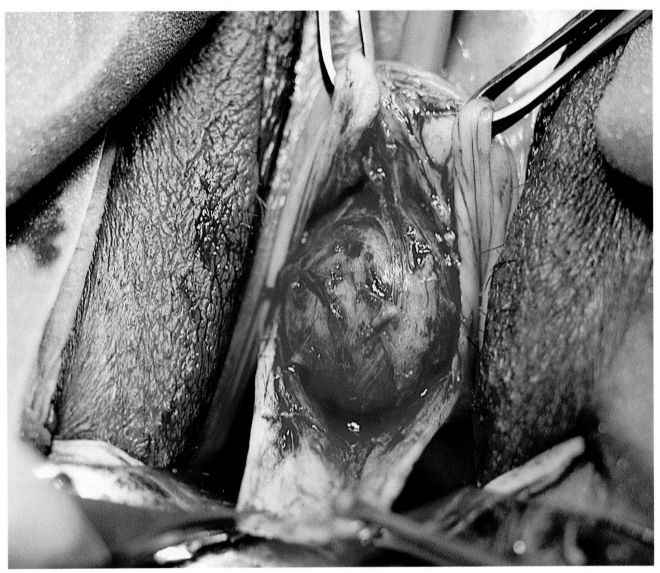

STEP 2:

An anterior vaginal wall flap is reflected posteriorly from the urethral meatus to the bladder neck, exposing the periurethral fascia. Care is taken to avoid any perforation or entry into this fascia or the diverticulum.

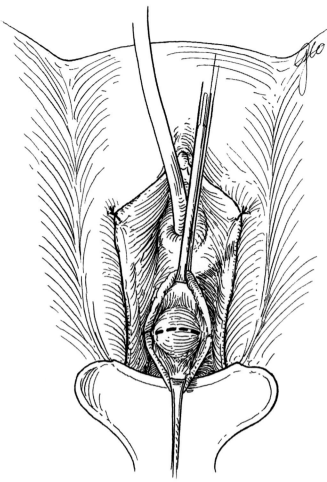

STEP 3:

The periurethral fascia and muscular wall of the urethra are incised transversely over the area of the diverticulum. This fascia may be found very attenuated in patients with large diverticula.

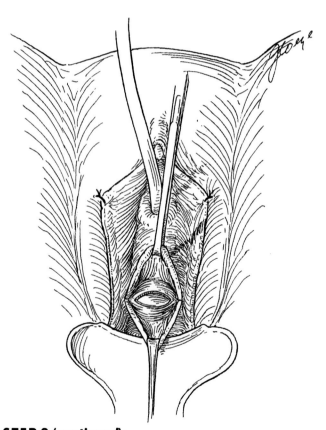

STEP 3 (*continued*):

Two flaps are created by dissection of the periurethral fascia proximally and distally to the incision. The spongy tissue of the submucosal layer of the urethral wall and the diverticular sac are exposed.

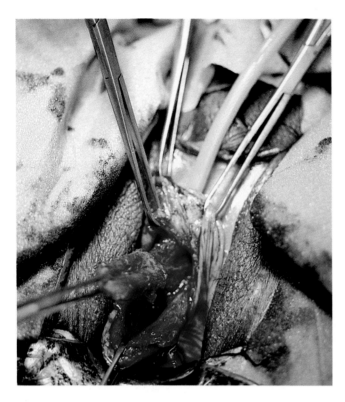

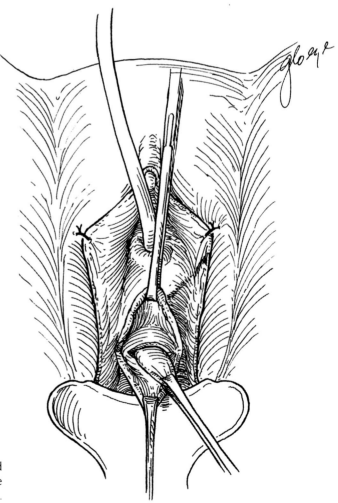

STEP 4:

Using sharp dissection, the wall of the diverticular sac is freed from the surrounding structures. The communication to the urethral lumen is isolated and excised flush to the urethral wall.

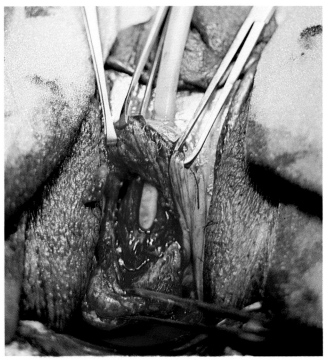

STEP 4 (continued):

In cases of severe inflammation, the sac may be very thin, adherent, and friable, requiring first the opening of the diverticulum and then excision of the sac.

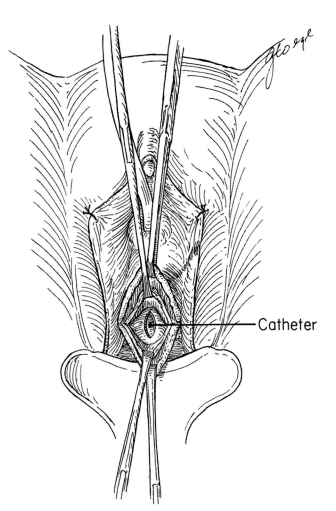

Catheter

STEP 4 (continued):

It is important that all the diverticular tissue and the urethral communication be completely excised. Very often a urethral mucosal defect and the indwelling catheter are seen.

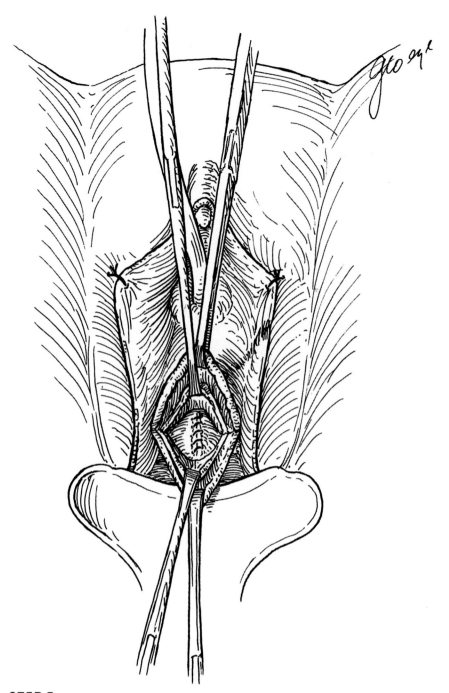

STEP 5:

The urethral wall is reconstructed by its anatomic layers. The mucosa and submucosal layers of the urethra are closed longitudinally with a running 3-0 absorbable suture over a 12 French catheter. The closure should be watertight and tension-free.

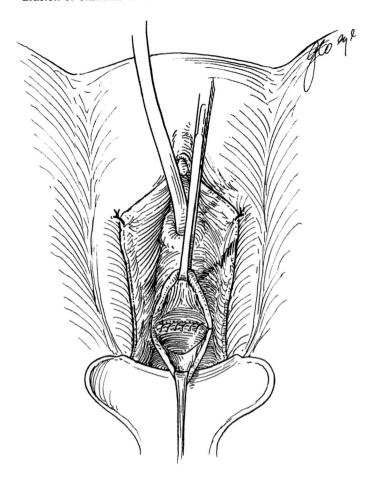

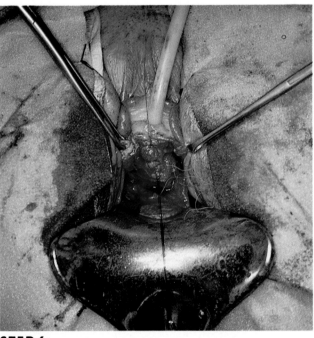

STEP 6:

The periurethral fascia is trimmed and closed horizontally, utilizing a 3-0 absorbable suture. This second layer of closure runs in a perpendicular direction with the first layer.

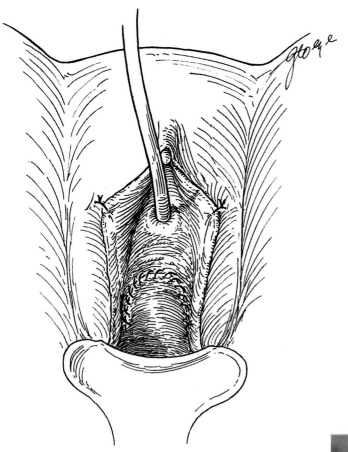

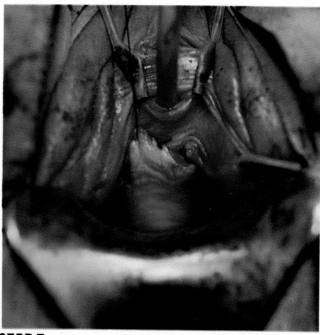

STEP 7:

The anterior vaginal wall flap is advanced and sutured well distal of the suture line of the periurethral fascia. The flap advancement brings fresh tissue to cover the reconstructed urethra as well and prevents overlapping lines of sutures.

After the procedure is completed, a vaginal pack is placed and the suprapubic and Foley catheters are connected to a drainage bag.

INTRAOPERATIVE COMPLICATIONS

Bleeding in the form of profuse oozing is not uncommon, particularly in patients with active infection and abscess formation. A vaginal packing should control this oozing.

It may be difficult to close the urethral mucosa, because the large defect created during the excision of the diverticulum may require further exposure of the urethral wall. We perform the closure over a 5 to 8 French feeding tube and have not encountered urethral strictures following this procedure.

In cases of difficult closure owing to severely inflamed or poor quality tissue, a fibrofatty labial (Martius) flap can be used between the periurethral fascia and the vaginal wall.

The finding of a large periurethral abscess may require a staged procedure, in which the abscess is drained and excision of the diverticulum performed as a secondary procedure.

A large proximal urethral diverticulum may extend into the trigone and bladder, or ureteric injury may occur. Instillation of indigo carmine into the bladder will assure bladder integrity, and cystoscopy after intravenous indigo carmine may be performed in selected cases to rule out ureteric injury.

POSTOPERATIVE CARE

Intravenous antibiotics are continued as indicated. The morning after operation, the packing is removed, and both catheters are attached with a Y connector to one bag. The patient may be discharged one or two days after operation. Three to seven days after surgery the urethral catheter is removed, and on days 10 to 14, a voiding cystogram is performed through the suprapubic catheter.

POSTOPERATIVE COMPLICATIONS

Prior to surgery, proper antibiotic therapy is mandatory. Reconstructive surgery in patients with active urinary and diverticular infection may lead to fistula formation and recurrent diverticula.

Important factors in operative success and avoidance of fistula formation include a watertight closure, precise dissection, and anatomic closure of the urethral layers, avoiding overlapping lines of suture. Urethrovaginal fistula formation is the most difficult complication of diverticular surgery and should be treated after a reasonable period of healing. Anterior vaginal infection is rare and responds well to antibiotics. If an abscess forms, surgical drainage is required in spite of the potential damage to the repair.

Urethral diverticula may recur, particularly in patients with active urethral infection, difficult dissection, or tension of the suture lines, and when postoperative difficulties with catheter drainage are encountered. Secondary surgery should be performed after a prudent period of observation.

Stress incontinence prior to surgery should be well documented and could be corrected in selected cases at the time of the excision of the diverticulum. Secondary urinary stress incontinence not present prior to surgical therapy is rare and may develop in patients with prior anatomic defects because of dissection of the urethral support. Severe incontinence caused by a nonfunctional sphincter may occur from extensive dissection of the urethral wall. Surgical therapy for this condition may require a sling procedure or periurethral injections.

TRANSVAGINAL

RECONSTRUCTION

OF THE FEMALE

URETHRA

Indications

Transvaginal repair of a damaged, nonfunctional urethra is one of the most challenging problems in vaginal surgery. Indications for surgery include congenital anomalies, damaged urethra due to multiple operations or radiation therapy, and pelvic trauma (Fig. 9–1). The urethra is anatomically short, open, fixed, and incompetent. The goals of surgical therapy include (a) creation of a continent sphincter mechanism, (b) construction of a conduit for the urine to flow in a normal vaginal location, and (c) covering the area with fresh, vascularized tissues to avoid fistula formation.

Diagnosis

The diagnosis of urethral damage is very simple. The clinical history is of severe incontinence after radiation, trauma, or multiple operations. The physical examination will reveal an open and short urethra with constant dribbling of urine. Sometimes only the bladder neck is intact and the rest of the urethra is necrotic or absent. A large urethral fistula may be present with a small distal or proximal segment of urethra still intact.

Evaluation prior to surgery should include cystoscopy and cystometry to rule out intravesical pathology and to assess functional bladder capacity.

Surgical Techniques

Two transvaginal techniques will be described: one includes rotating a flap of vaginal wall and the other is an in situ urethral reconstruction. An abdominovaginal urethral procedure is discussed in which the urethra is congenitally absent. In this patient the bladder was shaped into a tube to form a neourethra, and the bladder capacity was restored by enlargement cystoplasty.

Urethral Reconstruction by Vaginal Wall Flap Rotation

This reconstruction is preferred when the urethral length is shortened but the bladder neck and proximal urethra are intact. The rest of the anterior vaginal wall must have good tissue quality.

The main goal of surgery is to elongate the urethral canal, preventing voiding within the vagina. Continence is not restored by this procedure. If urethral hypermobility and stress incontinence are present, a needle bladder neck suspension could be performed simultaneously. In this case the suspension sutures are applied prior to the urethral reconstruction, and the sutures in the suprapubic area are left untied until the completion of the urethral procedure. If the bladder neck and proximal urethra are open, fixed, and incompetent (intrinsic sphincter dysfunction), a fascial sling procedure is strongly recommended.

The patient is in the lithotomy position. After preparation and draping, a suprapubic catheter and a small urethral Foley catheter (8 to 10 French) are inserted. Perioperative antibiotics are given.

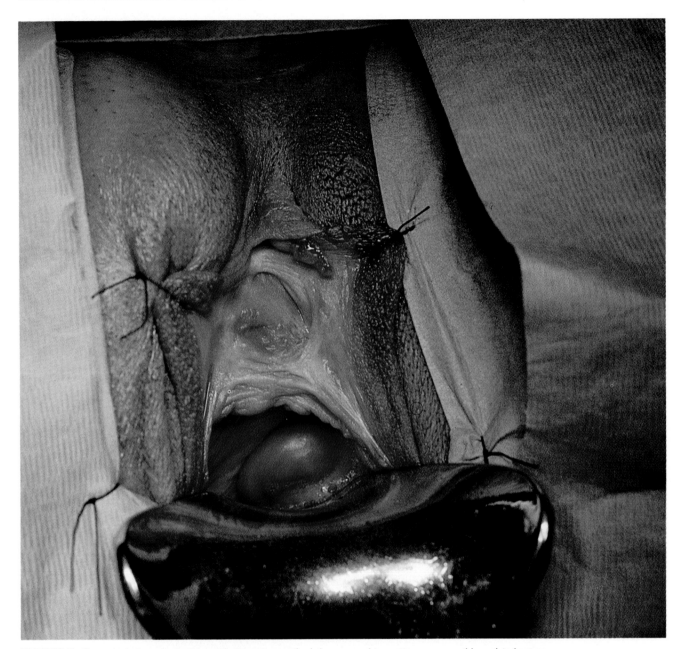

FIGURE 9–1. Vaginal view of a patient with extensive urethral damage and incontinence, caused by pelvic fracture.

SURGICAL TECHNIQUE

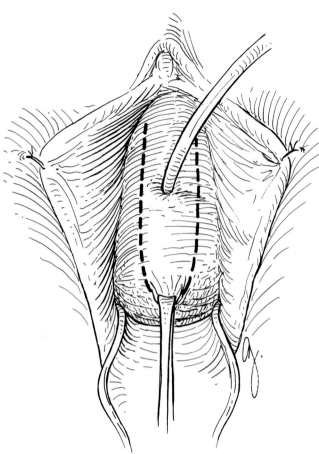

STEP 1:

With the urethral catheter under slight tension, the bladder neck area is outlined. A U-shaped incision is made in the intact vaginal wall 2 to 3 cm posterior to the bladder neck. The two parallel arms of the incision are extended at each side of the bladder neck or urethral opening toward the area of the future urethral meatus. Dissection is carried out laterally, undermining the vaginal wall 1 to 2 cm from the incision. In the distal segment the base of the labia is exposed, while in the proximal area the periurethral and perivesical fascia are uncovered.

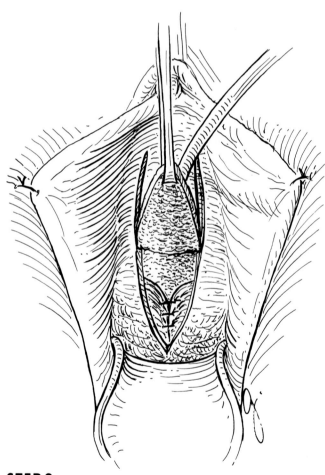

STEP 2:

A flap of vaginal wall is prepared with its base around the bladder neck or proximal urethra. Care is taken to preserve its blood supply. The flap is advanced around the urethral Foley catheter and toward the area selected as the new urethral meatus. Plication of the bladder neck is performed using 2-0 absorbable sutures.

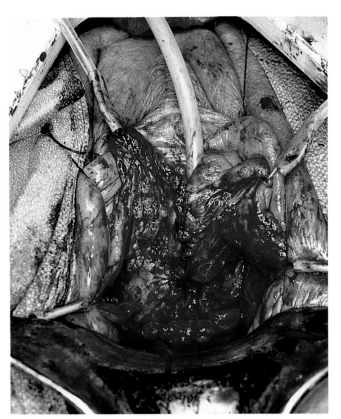

STEP 3:

Interrupted fine absorbable sutures are used to secure the edges of the flap to the medial margin of the vaginal incision, creating a urethral tube. If a sling procedure is going to be performed, the fascial strip is transferred at this time, underneath the bladder neck, and anchored with absorbable sutures to the perivesical fascia.

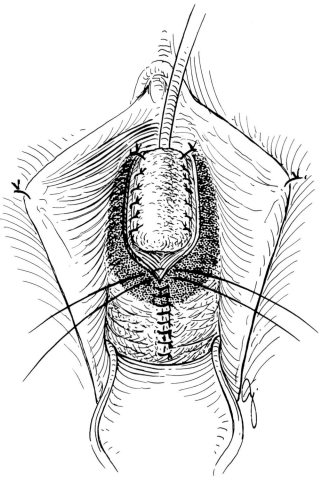

STEP 4:

Interrupted sutures are used to approximate the lateral edge of the vaginal incision in order to cover the neourethra and the fascial sling or Martius flap, if created.

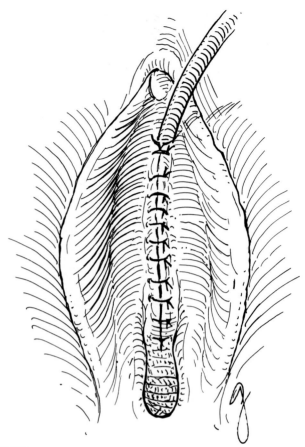

STEP 5:

Final view of the anterior vaginal wall after reconstruction. The external meatus is also fashioned with interrupted sutures.

IN SITU URETHRAL RECONSTRUCTION

This reconstruction is also performed in cases of extensive urethral damage (Fig. 9–2). It does not require flap advancement of the vaginal wall. The goal of in situ reconstruction is to restore the urethral length to normal, restore the external urethral meatus to a normal anatomic position, and provide continence. Concomitant or secondary procedures like a Martius fibrofatty graft, bladder neck suspension, bladder neck reconstruction, and fascial slings generally are required.

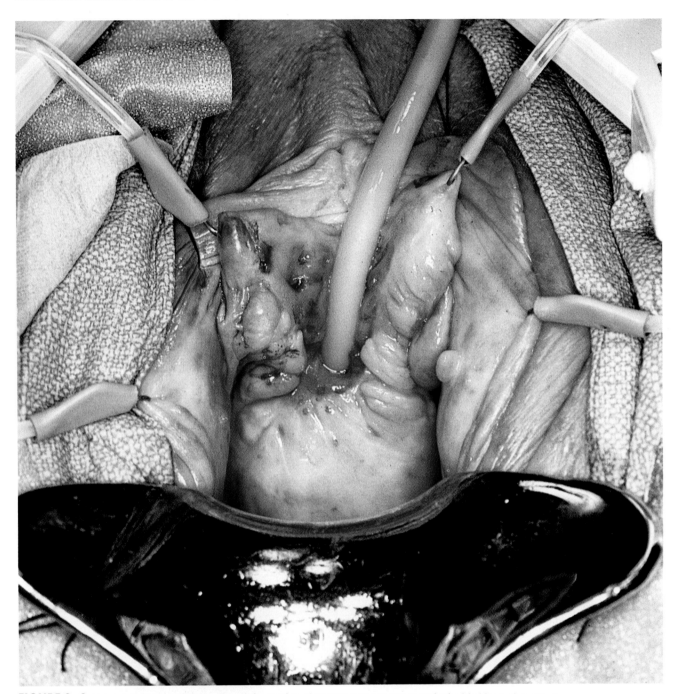

FIGURE 9—2. Extensive damage and necrosis of the urethra after prior anterior repair. Only the bladder neck is intact.

SURGICAL TECHNIQUE

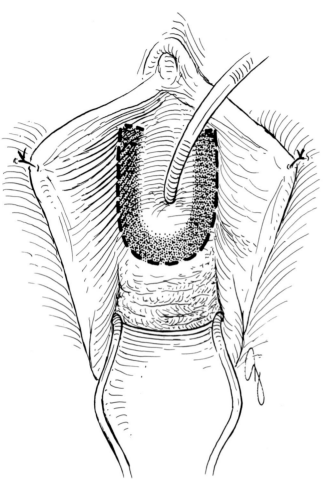

STEP 1:

A **U** incision is made around the remaining urethra or bladder neck. Dissection is carried out underneath the medial portion of the incision, undermining the vaginal wall.

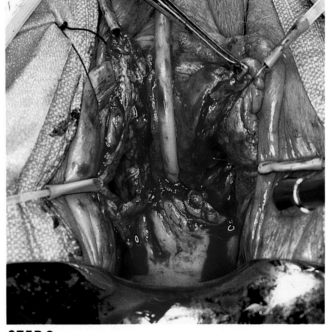

STEP 2:

The Foley catheter is aligned over the island of vagina wall. This tissue will be used as the first layer of the neourethra.

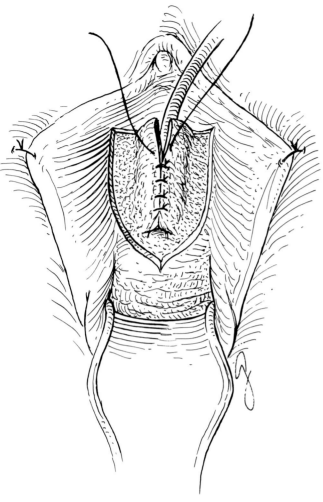

STEP 3:

Reconstruction of the urethral canal is initiated by rolling the medial edges of the incision over a small (8 to 10 French) urethral catheter. Fine, interrupted 4-0 absorbable sutures are used to approximate the vaginal wall to the midline.

Bladder neck reconstruction is performed by excising a triangular wedge of bladder neck and trigone. The ureteric orifices must be visualized or catheterized if required. Interrupted mattress sutures of the bladder wall are used to approximate the free edges of the trigonal area and bladder neck. The sutures are tied snug over the small urethral catheter, providing mucosa-to-mucosa approximation of the lumen and a strong and thick smooth muscle envelope. At least 1.5 to 2 cm of bladder neck elongation should be obtained.

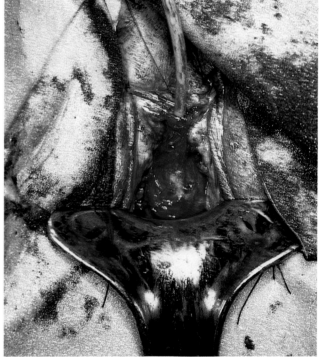

STEP 4:

The first layer of the urethral reconstruction has been completed, obtaining a 3-cm anatomic length of urethra. A fascial sling will be used to support and provide coaptation to the neourethra.

STEP 5:

If a fibrofatty labial graft is indicated, it should be retrieved at this stage. The graft should cover the entire length of the urethra.

If a sling procedure will be performed simultaneously, the periurethral area is dissected free and the retropubic space is entered to free any retropubic adhesions. A 15 × 2 cm segment of anterior abdominal wall fascia is retrieved, and its ends are anchored with a helix of Number 1 Prolene suture. Using a long hemostatic clamp and under finger control in the retropubic space, the tip of the clamp is transferred from the suprapubic to the vaginal area. The ends of the Prolene sutures are transferred from the vaginal to the suprapubic area. The fascial sling is secured to the first layer of the reconstructed urethra with interrupted absorbable sutures. The free ends of the Prolene sutures are left untied over the suprapubic area until the vaginal wall closure is completed.

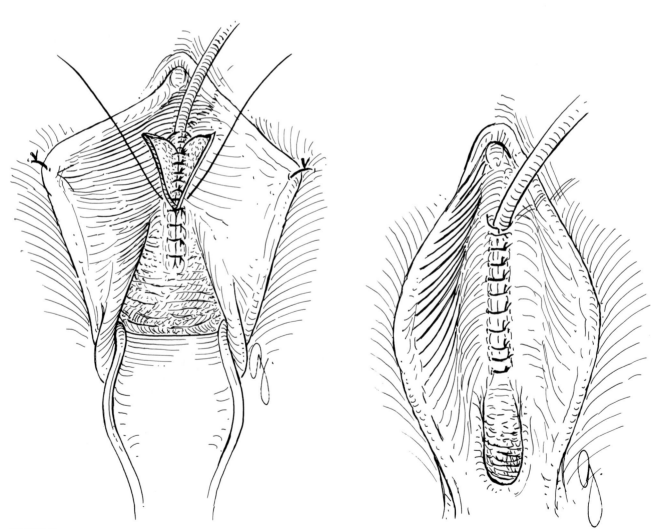

STEP 6:

Final closure of the vaginal wall covering the sling and/or the fibrofatty labial pad. The lateral margins of the original incision are undermined and approximated with interrupted sutures to the midline. Tension should be avoided. The new external meatus is reconstructed. A vaginal packing is inserted into the vagina.

Intraoperative Complications

Complications do not differ from those of other vaginal procedures. Bleeding can be more prominent due to multiple prior operations. Extensive tissue loss may make it difficult to cover the vaginal wall after completion of the urethral tubularization. In this case a rotational flap of the labia with its underlying fibrofatty tissue can be used to provide proper cover. Proper ureteric visualization and catheterization are very important in avoiding ureter injury.

Postoperative Complications

The two main complications of this procedure are urethrovaginal fistula and urinary incontinence. Fistula formation can be prevented by avoiding tension of the suture lines, proper tissue mobilization, infection prevention, and judicious use of the fibrofatty labial fat. After a proper healing period the fistula can be repaired transvaginally. Incontinence of urine may result from poor coaptation and atrophy of the neourethra. Using small urethral catheters for a short time, good tissue apposition, and avoiding tension on sutures should create a competent and functional urethra. Injections of collagen or Teflon can be used in patients with recurrent incontinence to improve the seal effect of the urethra.

ABDOMINOVAGINAL URETHRAL RECONSTRUCTION

In selected cases of absent urethra due to congenital (Figs. 9–3 and 9–4), traumatic, or surgical reasons, part of the bladder may be used to create a neourethra. The bladder must be compliant, not be radiated, and have a good vascular supply. The small functional bladder capacity will be restored to normal by enlargement cystoplasty.

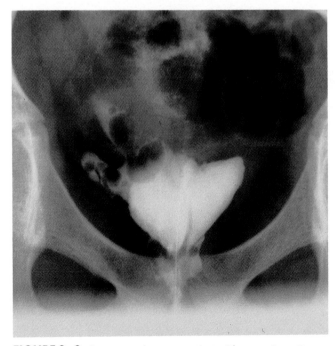

FIGURE 9–3. Cystogram of a young patient with severe incontinence due to congenital absence of the urethra.

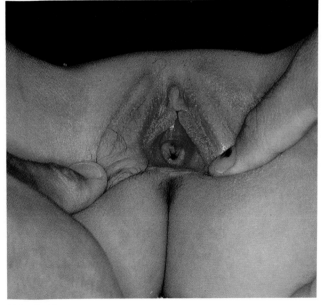

FIGURE 9–4. Vaginal examination showing the bladder neck at the anterior vaginal wall.

SURGICAL TECHNIQUE

STEP 1:

The patient is in the low lithotomy position, exposing the lower abdomen and vagina. A transverse suprapubic incision is made, and the retropubic space is exposed. The bladder neck is dissected free from the perivaginal fascia and disconnected from its vaginal communication. The vaginal wall is closed except in the most distal area, where a tunnel is created to accommodate the neourethra. The abdominovaginal approach facilitates the creation of this tunnel. Transvaginally placed interrupted sutures anchor the edges of the vaginal wall of this opening, the future location of the new external urethral meatus.

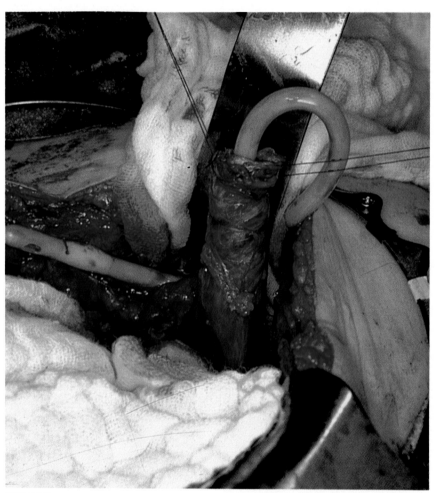

STEP 2:

The neourethra has been created from an anterior bladder wall flap. The ureters are visualized, catheterized, and secured with sutures. Two parallel incisions are made in the anterior bladder wall, 4 to 5 cm long and 2 cm wide, isolating a well-vascularized rectangular flap. A small Foley catheter (8 to 10 French) is used. Two-layer closure of the bladder flap will be performed, using a running and a second interrupted line of sutures. The Foley catheter is secured to the neourethra and its balloon inflated.

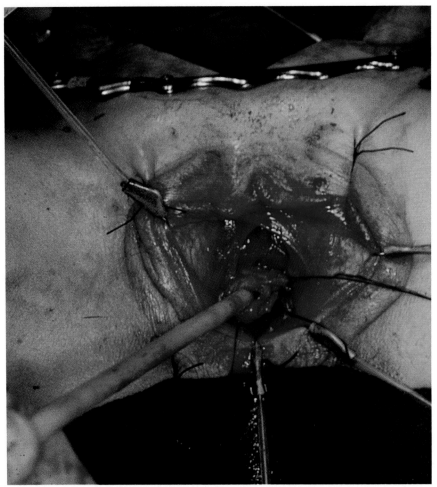

STEP 3:

The tip of a long hemostatic clamp is transferred from the vagina to the retropubic space through the previously opened tract. The end of the clamp grasps the urethral catheter and its anchoring sutures, transferring the end of the neourethra to the vaginal area. Interrupted sutures are used to anchor the vaginal wall to the bladder tube. A vaginal packing is left in the vagina.

STEP 4:

The retropubic part of the surgery will be completed. If bladder capacity is acceptable, the surgery is completed after insertion of a suprapubic catheter. If the bladder capacity is very small (organic or functional), an enlargement cystoplasty should be performed. A segment of ileum or cecum is isolated and the bowel reanastomosed. The selected loop of bowel is detubularized and anastomosed to the open bladder. If the reconstructed urethra requires a procedure for stabilization and compression by a sling or suspension procedure, this should be completed at this time. The abdomen is closed after placement of drains in the retropubic space.

TRANSVAGINAL

CLOSURE OF THE

BLADDER NECK

INDICATIONS

Extensive urethral destruction is one of the recognized complications of a long-term indwelling urethral catheter. Damage to the urethral wall results from pressure necrosis of the catheter and self-retaining balloon and from spontaneous extrusion due to bladder spasms. Larger and larger catheters are used until progressive distention results in urethral destruction and incontinence around the catheter. Closure of the bladder neck and permanent suprapubic catheter insertion are indicated in patients whose poor general condition rules against a major reconstruction. Transvaginal closure of the bladder neck is generally used in conjunction with reconstructive bladder procedures, such as continent enlargement cystoplasty.

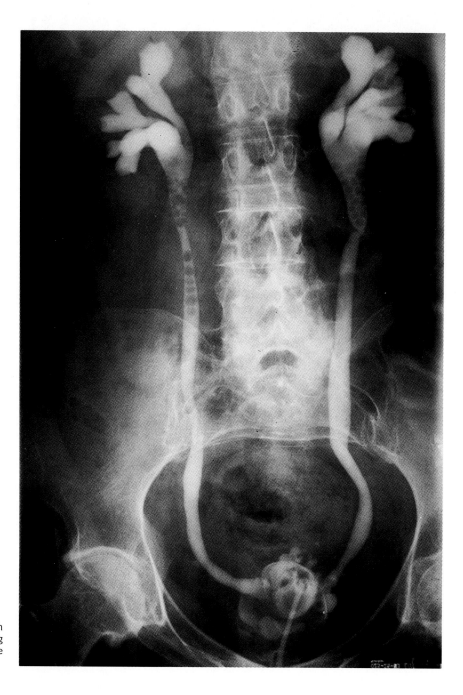

FIGURE 10–1. Cystogram of a patient with severe, progressive multiple sclerosis, showing bilateral reflux and incontinence around the Foley catheter.

DIAGNOSIS

The clinical history generally reveals urinary incontinence around a long-term indwelling Foley catheter. Usually, increasingly large catheters have been used to overcome the incontinence. On physical examination the urethral meatus is very patulous, the urethra is shortened, and the bladder neck sometimes can be visualized during inspection of the urethra. Cystoscopy is carried out to verify the absence of other pathology, mainly neoplastic changes in the bladder as a result of prolonged irritation by the indwelling catheter (Figs. 10–1 and 10–2).

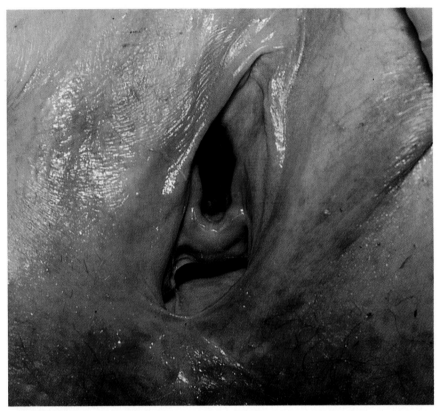

FIGURE 10–2. Destroyed urethra and wide-open bladder neck due to the chronic indwelling catheter in the patient shown in Figure 10–1.

SURGICAL TECHNIQUE

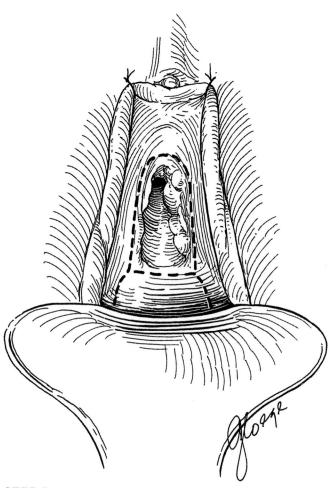

STEP 1:

With the patient in a dorsal lithotomy position, the lower abdomen and vagina are prepped and draped in sterile fashion. The labia are retracted laterally with stay sutures, and a weighted posterior vaginal retractor is inserted. A suprapubic cystostomy tube, usually a 22 French Foley catheter, is positioned in the bladder (see Chapter 3 for placement of a cystostomy tube using the curved Lowsley retractor).

After normal saline is injected into the anterior vaginal wall, an incision is made circumscribing the destroyed urethra; it is extended by an inverted **U** incision in the anterior vaginal wall.

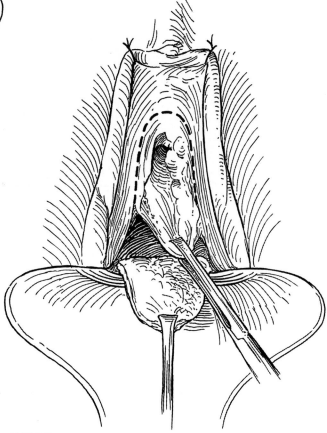

STEP 2:

A vaginal flap is created by sharp dissection of the anterior vaginal wall from the underlying perivesical fascia. The dissection is extended around the open bladder neck.

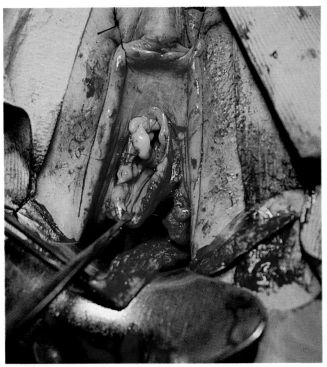

STEP 3:

The dissection around the bladder neck is advanced laterally toward the rami of the pubic bone. As in needle bladder neck suspension surgery (see Chapter 5), the urethropelvic fascia is entered sharply on either side of the bladder neck, freeing the bladder from its attachments to the pubic bone and lateral pelvic wall.

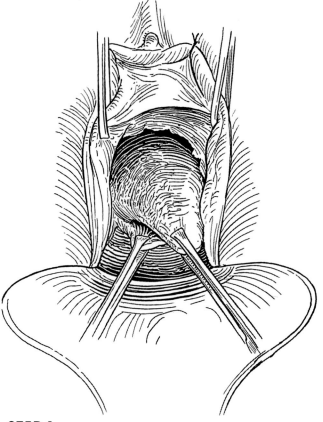

STEP 4:

The pubourethral ligaments are transected to allow complete mobilization of the bladder outlet from the symphysis pubis.

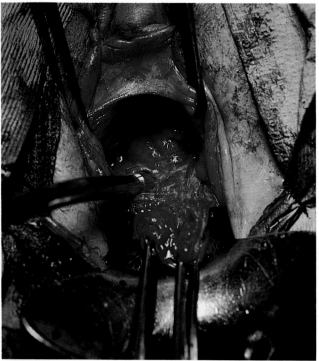

STEP 5:

Indigo carmine is injected intravenously to facilitate identification of the ureteral orifices and their relationship to the bladder neck. The remnants of the scarred proximal urethra are excised, avoiding any injury to the ureteral orifices.

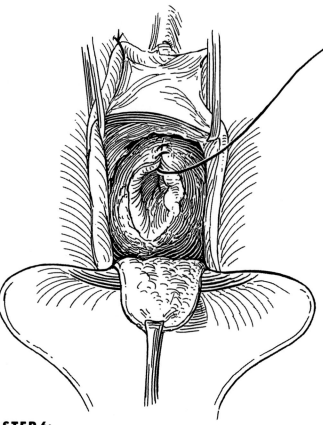

STEP 6:

The bladder neck is closed in a vertical and anteroposterior direction with a running 2-0 polyglycolic acid suture.

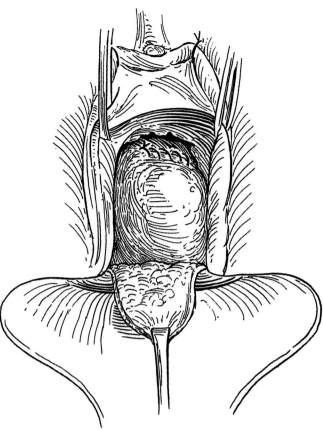

STEP 6 (*continued*):

A second layer of interrupted 2-0 polyglycolic acid suture is placed. This suture line includes the bladder neck and the anterior bladder wall, just behind the symphysis pubis. This maneuver allows the transfer of the underlying closed bladder neck to the retropubic space, high behind the symphysis pubis.

A small incision is made in the suprapubic area, a large clamp is transferred under finger control to the vaginal area, and a Penrose drain is positioned in the retropubic space.

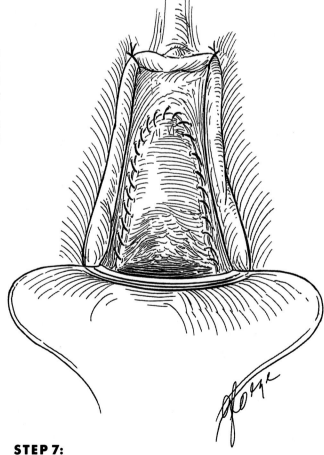

STEP 7:

The anterior vaginal flap is advanced as a third layer to cover the previous urethral opening.

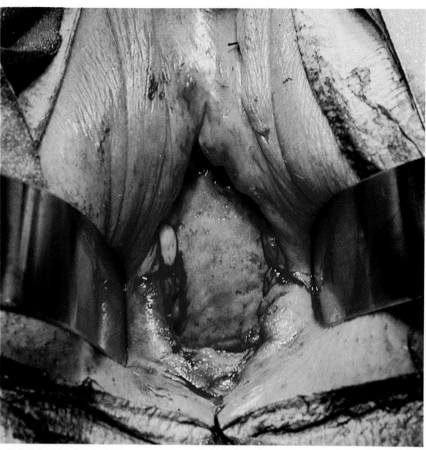

STEP 7 (*continued*):

A running 2-0 polyglycolic acid suture is used to suture the margin of the anterior vaginal wall. If needed, a Martius flap may be interposed before the vaginal advancement is done.

POSTOPERATIVE CARE

Infection is prevented by preoperative antibiotic therapy. Bleeding is minimal, of short duration, and easily controlled by the vaginal packing. The suprapubic tube is irrigated frequently to verify proper drainage and connected to a closed bag drainage until adequate healing has been obtained. It is then changed at intervals of 2 to 3 weeks.

POSTOPERATIVE COMPLICATIONS

The most worrisome complication is a vesicovaginal fistula. The surgical details that are vital for prevention of this complication include (1) complete mobilization of the bladder outlet from the pubic bone attachments; (2) positioning of the closed bladder neck high behind the symphysis pubis; (3) advancement of a vaginal flap to cover the underlying layers without apposition of the suture lines; (4) use of a retropubic Penrose drain; and (5) use of a Martius flap when necessary. Retropubic bleeding or infection may require surgical drainage.

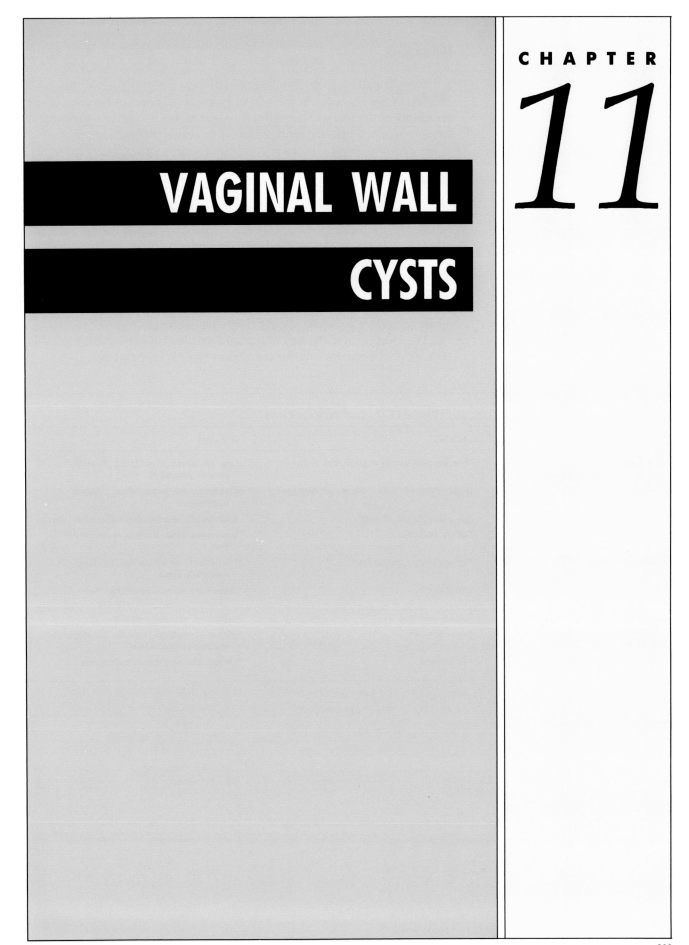

VAGINAL WALL
CYSTS

INDICATIONS

Vaginal wall cysts are uncommon and have differing causes. The presence of a painless mass in the vagina is always of concern because of the possibility of carcinoma. Operation is indicated if the mass is symptomatic, fast-growing, and creating pain or urinary or sexual dysfunction.

DIAGNOSIS

The history is in general nonspecific. In most cases, the cyst is discovered incidentally during routine vaginal examination. The mass is not tender, if not infected; it is cystic, mobile, and well defined. Any other findings must be recorded, such as stress incontinence or cystocele that may rerquire concomitant therapy. Imaging by ultrasound, computed tomography, or magnetic resonance is rarely necessary but may help delineate the extent of the lesion. Cystogram, intravenous pyelogram, and cystoscopy may help define an ectopic ureterocele. Carcinoma should always be ruled out.

The location and etiology of vaginal cystic lesions are outlined in Table 11–1. Several cystic lesions are pictured in Figures 11–1 through 11–6.

TABLE 11–1. VAGINAL WALL CYSTS		
Diagnosis	**Location**	**Histology**
Gartner cyst	Anterior and lateral vaginal wall	Low columnar, nonciliated. Smooth muscle around it
Adenosis	Upper third of vagina. Single or multiple	Columnar, mucin-secreting, ciliated epithelium
Endometriosis	Any place. Cyclic changes	Endometrial glands. Blue-chocolate cyst
Keratinous or epidermoid cyst	Mainly posterior	Squamous cells. No mucus. Inclusion cyst
Diverticulum	Periurethral. Anterior wall	Transitional or squamous. Urethral communication
Minor vestibular gland (Skene)	Distal urethra	Columnar, mucous secretion. No communication with urethra
Bartholin cyst	Lateral introitus	Columnar, mucous secretion
Urethral prolapse	Distal urethra	Hernia of urethral mucosa. Transitional/ squamous epithelium
Ectopic ureterocele	Periurethral	Transitional/squamous epithelium

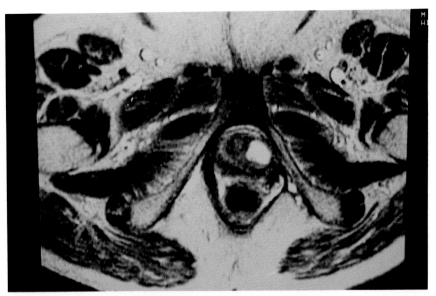

FIGURE 11—1. Magnetic resonance imaging of the urethral area in a patient with a tender anterior vaginal wall mass. The final diagnosis was periurethral cyst.

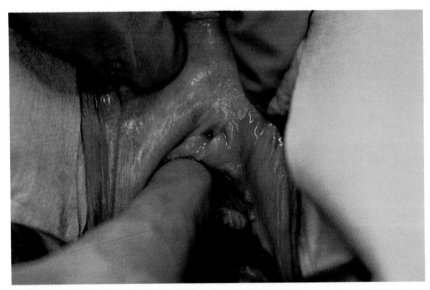

FIGURE 11—2. Small distal Skene gland cyst, with purulent drainage, in a patient with recurrent urinary tract infection.

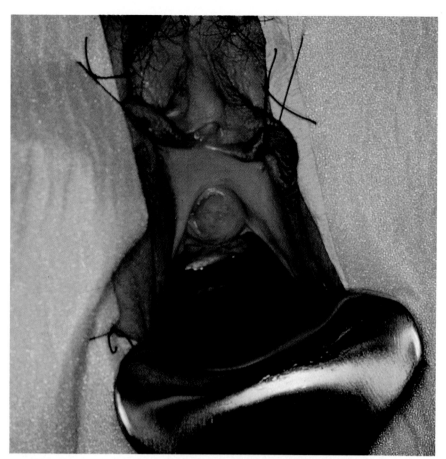

FIGURE 11–3. Large periurethral cyst causing urinary obstructive symptoms.

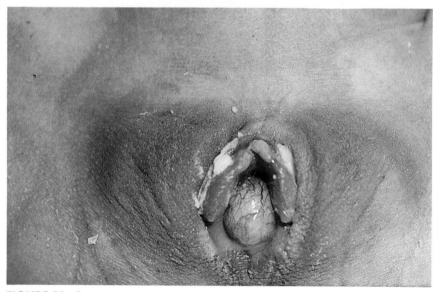

FIGURE 11–4. Cystic periurethral lesion confirmed to be an ectopic ureterocele.

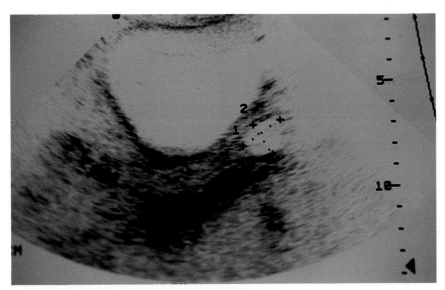

FIGURE 11–5. Transvaginal ultrasound study in a patient suffering from vaginal pain, frequency, and urgency. A cystic lesion is well defined posterior to the bladder.

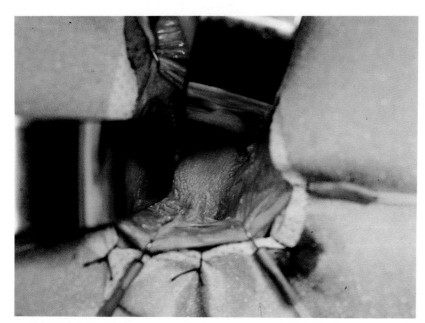

FIGURE 11–6. Vaginal examination of the patient shown in Figure 11–5, revealing a cystic lesion in the posterolateral aspect of the vagina. Excision of the cyst was performed; the lesion was found to be a Gartner cyst.

A.   EXCISION OF BARTHOLIN CYST

INDICATIONS FOR SURGERY

Symptoms of a mass, difficulties with pain, and dyspareunia are indications for surgery. If the initial presentation is of an abscess, drainage and marsupialization of the cyst are performed.

SURGICAL TECHNIQUE

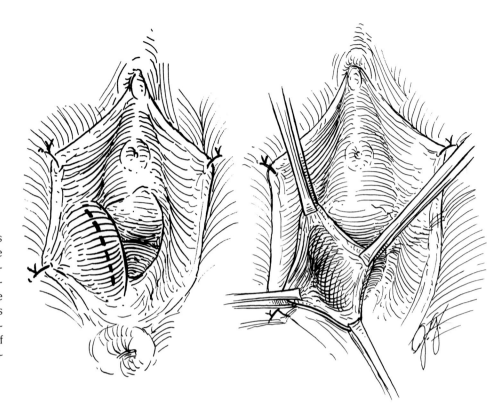

STEP 1:

Lateral labial retraction is achieved with silk sutures. The cyst is elevated by gentle pressure from behind in the genitofemoral sulcus with the assistant's hand. Incision is made through the lateral vaginal wall at the medial aspect of the labium minus longitudinally.

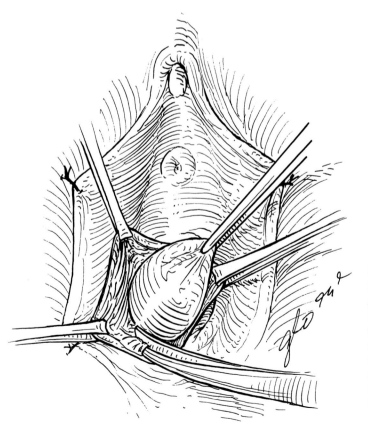

STEP 2:

Beginning at the lower part of the cyst, skin edges are grasped with delicate clamps, and the cyst is mobilized from the surrounding tissues using blunt and sharp dissection with Metzenbaum scissors. Bleeding is kept to a minimum by staying as close to the cyst wall as possible and using cautery as needed. Dissection of the lower pole will require occasional placement of a gloved finger in the rectum to gauge distance, as glandular parenchyma may be in close proximity.

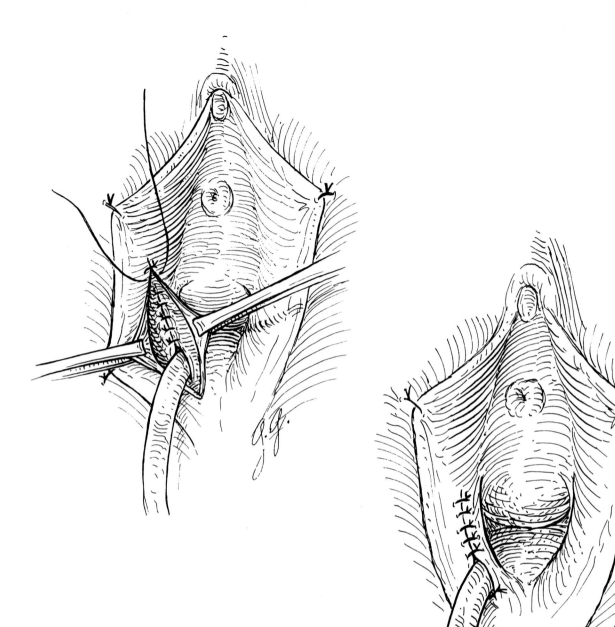

STEP 3:

After mobilization of the lower pole of the cyst, dissection continues on to the upper pole. Here, dissection is made easier by gentle forward traction on the cyst wall with grasping forceps. Glandular parenchyma may extend far upward beneath the bulbocavernosus muscle, and dissection is assisted by frequent use of hemostatic clamps to assure a dry field of vision. Once all remaining glandular elements are removed, the cavity is irrigated and complete hemostasis is achieved. Vicryl 3-0 is then utilized for a multilayered closure of the defect. If complete hemostasis cannot be completely assured, drainage with a Penrose drain for 24 hours should be instituted.

INTRAOPERATIVE COMPLICATIONS

Severe hemorrhage from the adjacent vestibular bulb may occur, especially if dissection is started at the upper pole of the cyst. Freeing the lower pole first provides an attached pedicle to aid in retraction and dissection as well as leaving the more vascular upper pole for last. Bladder, urethral, and rectal injury can occur.

POSTOPERATIVE CARE

If no infection is present, the patient may be discharged from the recovery room provided all vital signs have been stable, and she feels comfortable. Oral antibiotics and sitz baths are taken for the first postoperative week.

POSTOPERATIVE COMPLICATIONS

Insufficient hemostasis can lead to a massive hematoma in the wound cavity if a drain has not been left in place. If any portions of the cyst wall and glandular parenchyma are left in situ, recurrence is the rule. Furthermore, if the cyst cavity has been entered in the course of dissection, the margins of the resected cyst will be difficult to remove entirely and recurrence can be expected.

B. MARSUPIALIZATION OF BARTHOLIN CYST

INDICATIONS FOR SURGERY

Surgical therapy is indicated for dyspareunia, chronic vaginal discomfort, secondary infection, and voiding difficulties from urethral or bladder neck obstruction.

DIAGNOSIS

A clinical history of vaginal discomfort, dyspareunia, or obstructive voiding symptoms is obtained. Physical examination discloses a Bartholin cyst in the usual location—the lateral introitus just medial to the labia minora. It may encompass the entire lateral vaginal wall in this location or it may be seen as a discrete, circumscribed protuberance. When secondarily infected, the cyst is converted to a pseudoabscess with surrounding vaginal mucosal inflammation.

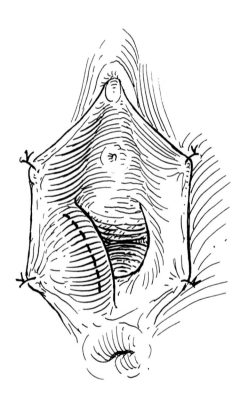

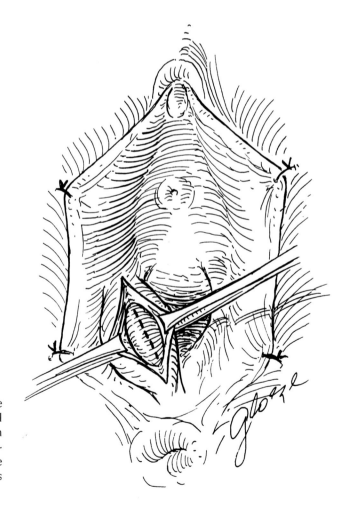

STEP 1:

Lateral labial retraction is achieved with silk sutures, and the cyst is elevated by pressure from behind in the genitofemoral sulcus with the assistant's hand. An incision is made through the vaginal wall over the protruding cyst in a longitudinal direction, and the cyst cavity itself is then opened over its entire length. The thick mucus within the cyst cavity (or pus if it has been secondarily infected) is then drained.

SURGICAL TECHNIQUE

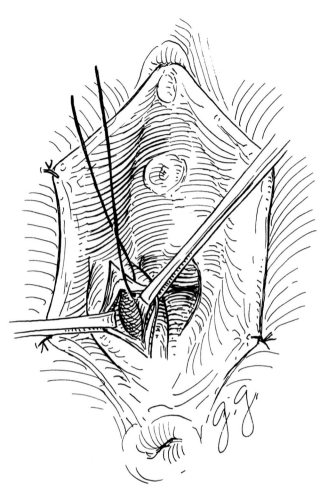

STEP 2:

Using 2-0 Vicryl, the cut edges of the wall are approximated to surrounding vaginal wall. If the procedure is performed in the presence of a Bartholin abscess, approximation will be difficult owing to the inflammation and edema of the surrounding vaginal wall. In this situation, larger, more encompassing stitches will be needed.

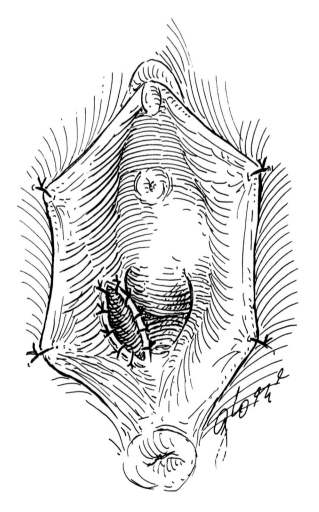

STEP 3:

The cavity is irrigated, and complete hemostasis is achieved. An antibiotic-soaked packing is then placed within the defect.

Intraoperative Complications

Possible complications at the time of surgery, such as bleeding, bladder or urethral perforation, or rectal injury, are very rare with this procedure.

Postoperative Care

If no infection is present, the patient may be discharged from the recovery room provided all vital signs have been stable, and she feels comfortable. Wound care is routine. The packing is removed on the first postoperative day. Oral antibiotics and sitz baths are taken for the first postoperative week.

Postoperative Complications

The cyst may recur, especially if the opening in the cyst was made too small and the entire length of the gland was not incised. An incision made too far laterally in the vestibular mucosa will lead to a poor cosmetic result as well as mucus production by the gland draining outside the vestibule.

C. EXCISION OF SKENE GLAND CYST

INDICATIONS

Recurrent urinary tract infection not responding to therapy, dyspareunia, obstructive urinary symptoms, and recurrent urethral discharge are some of the surgical indications. Therapeutic options include not only excision of the cyst but also aspiration (which increases the incidence of recurrence) and marsupialization of the cyst to the vaginal wall, avoiding the need for excision.

SURGICAL TECHNIQUE

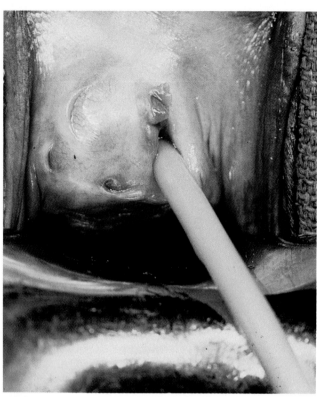

STEP 1:

A Foley catheter is inserted into the bladder after preparation and draping of the perineum and vaginal area.

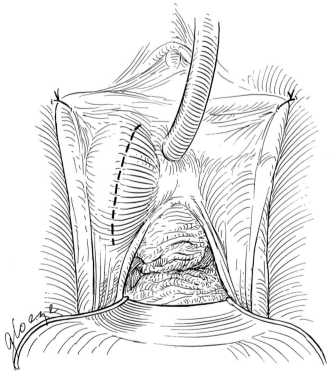

STEP 1 (*continued*):

An oblique incision is made over the cyst. The dissection is carried out around the pericystic tissue.

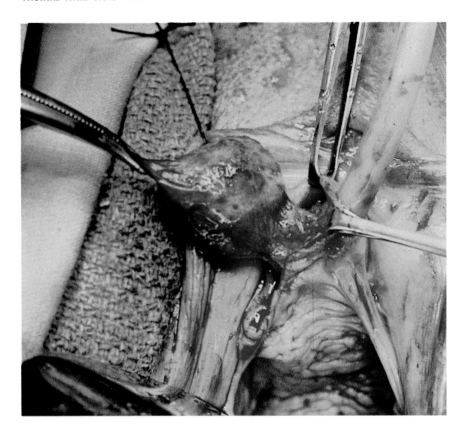

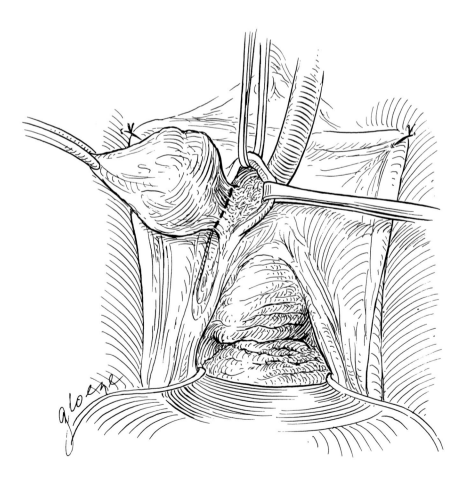

STEP 2:
The cyst is dissected free, exposing the occluded communication to the distal urethral meatus.

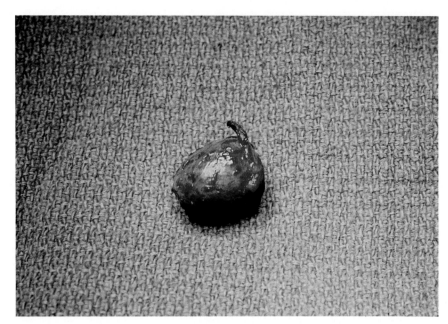

STEP 2 (continued):
The cyst has been excised completely, and its urethral communication is seen.

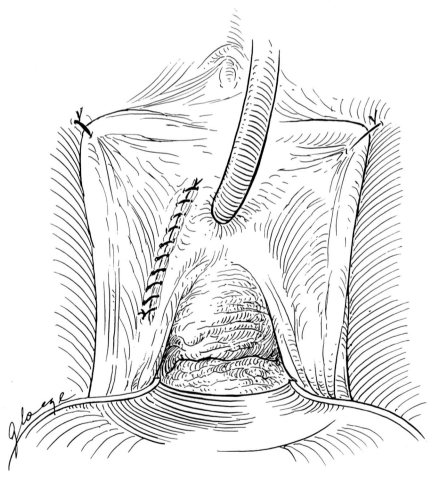

STEP 3:
The vaginal wall is closed. No drainage is required.

EXCISION

OF INFECTED

SKENE GLAND

INDICATIONS

In symptomatic patients with recurrent Skene gland infections that are unresponsive to long-term or differing courses of antibiotics and in whom other symptomatic therapy has failed, excision of the infected gland may be indicated. This situation is very rare now because of modern antibiotic therapy.

DIAGNOSIS

The patient gives a history of recurrent urinary tract infections and urethral pain. On physical examination a clear discharge of pus is seen from the Skene glands (Figs. 12–1 and 12–2). No collection or cyst is found, and the rest of the urethral examination is normal. Cystoscopy and cystogram are normal. Proper antibiotic therapy should be initiated for chronic suppression, if indicated. The patient must be re-examined after this period. In the rare cases in which this therapy fails and pus continues to be excreted at the urethral meatus, surgical therapy is necessary.

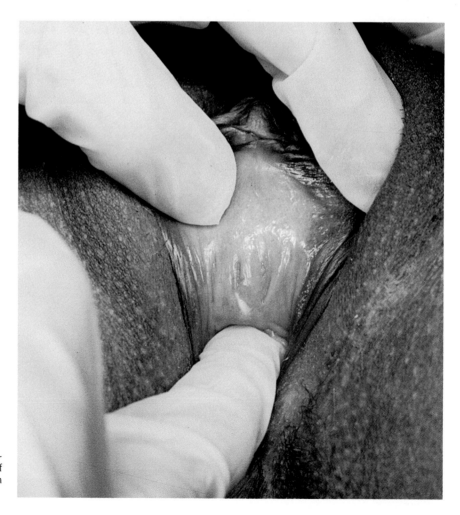

FIGURE 12–1. At vaginal examination, expression of the distal urethra shows drainage of pus through the opening of Skene glands on the right.

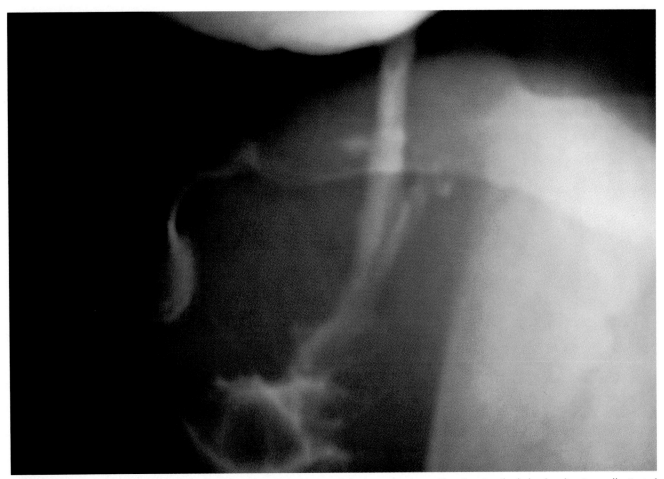

FIGURE 12—2. Voiding urethrogram in a patient with recurrent urinary infections, showing a dilated periurethral gland ending in a collection of contrast material.

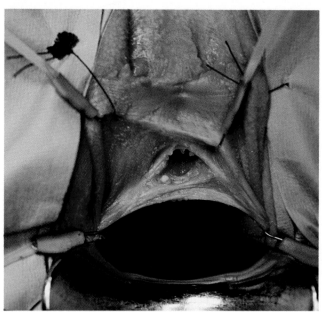

STEP 1:

Examination under anesthesia of the open urethral meatus shows pus draining from the Skene gland.

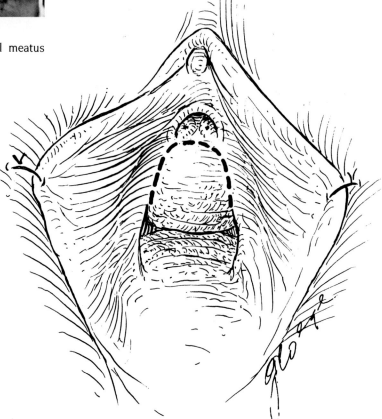

STEP 2:

With the patient in the lithotomy position, the vagina is prepared and draped in sterile fashion. A Foley catheter is inserted in the bladder. An Allis clamp is used to grasp the posterior lip of the external urethral meatus. A small, semicircular incision of the vaginal wall is made just proximal to the meatus.

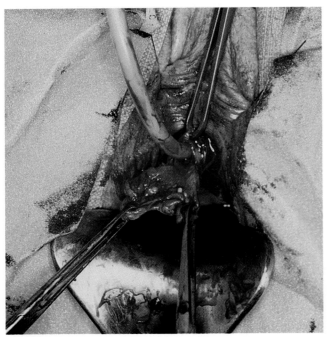

STEP 3:

After the flap is dissected free, a wedge resection of the posterior distal urethra is performed. The excision of 1 cm or less includes the entire urethral wall, periurethral tissue, and the Skene gland openings.

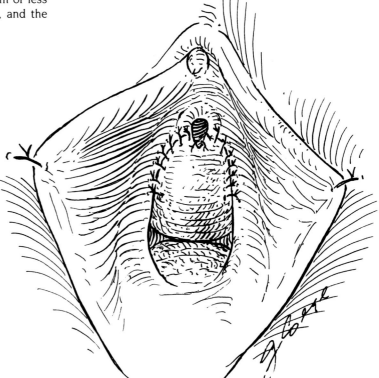

STEP 4:

The flap of vaginal wall is advanced forward. Interrupted fine absorbable sutures are used to approximate the vaginal wall to the urethral incision. The urethral meatus is now larger, slightly hypospadic, and elliptical.

A Foley catheter and a vaginal dressing are left in the vagina for 2 to 3 hours. This operation is performed as an outpatient procedure, with the patient discharged on oral antibiotics. Pain or other complications are very rare with this operation.

SEPARATION OF

LABIAL FUSION

INDICATIONS

Labial fusion is a congenital abnormality of the urogenital sinus. The labia majora are fused, covering the normal vaginal canal and urethra. As in cases of ambiguous genitalia, complete studies of the lower urinary tract and genital tract, as well as cytogenetic studies, should be performed. Surgical success indeed depends on proper evaluation and surgical indication.

With the patient under general anesthesia, endoscopy of the sinus is performed. A normal urethra and vagina are visualized underneath the fused skin.

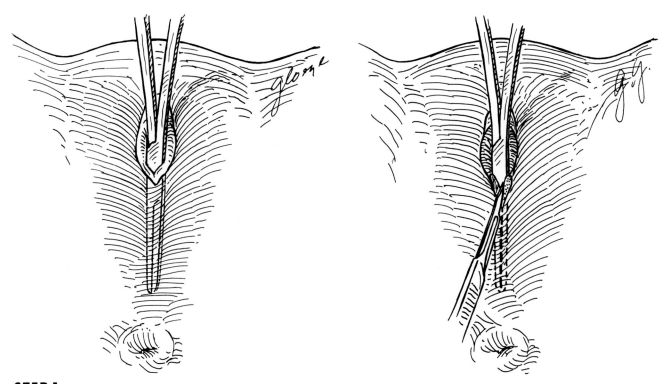

STEP 1:

A grooved sound or a small hemostatic clamp is inserted into the vagina. With forward traction, the skin is incised toward the perineum.

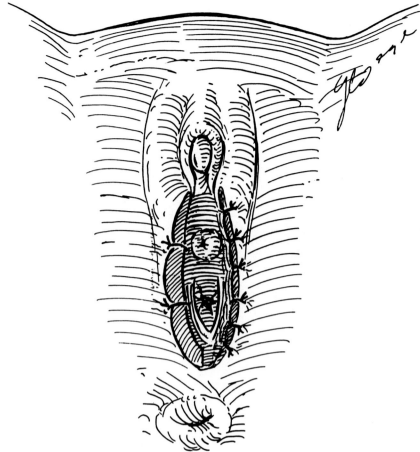

STEP 2:

The edges of the incision are sutured with fine absorbable sutures.

COMPLICATIONS

Complications of this procedure are very rare. The incision should be done with great care so as not to injure the rectum or urethra. Bleeding is controlled with fine, absorbable sutures.

EXCISION

OF URETHRAL

CARUNCLE

INDICATIONS

Atrophic changes of the vaginal wall and urethra may lead to urethral caruncle formation, a condition very common in elderly people. Recurrent bleeding, pain, recurrent urinary tract infection, and obstructive symptoms may be associated with urethral caruncle. Surgical therapy for this condition is very rarely required. Only symptomatic patients (with prolapse of the mucosa and obstructed symptoms) who do not respond to estrogens or local treatment are candidates for surgery.

DIAGNOSIS

The diagnosis is made by simple inspection of the external urethral meatus. A reddish, friable, inflamed urethral mucosa is often seen. Carcinoma of the distal urethra may present in a similar fashion, and biopsy should be done if required. As noted, the majority of patients do not require any therapy.

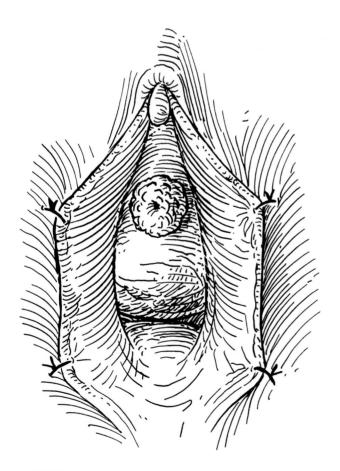

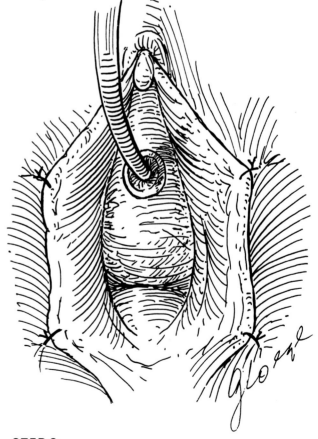

STEP 1:

With the patient in the lithotomy position, after preparation and draping, an Allis clamp grasps the end of the caruncle.

STEP 2:

A circumferential incision is made at the base of the lesion.

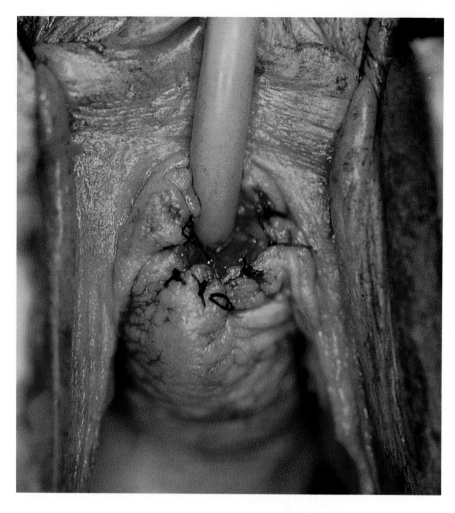

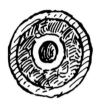

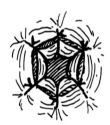

STEP 3:

After excision of the caruncle, fine absorbable sutures are applied between the urethral mucosa and vestibular epithelium. A Foley catheter is not required.

CONSTRUCTION

OF NEOVAGINA

Indications

Reconstruction of the vagina is indicated in cases of congenital absence (Fig. 15–1), various intersex conditions, trauma, and radiation injury and in patients undergoing ablative surgery for pelvic malignancy. The procedure may be performed in one stage after completion of a planned anterior exenteration.

Diagnosis

The diagnosis of vaginal agenesis is very simple. Pelvic ultrasound and urinary tract evaluation should be performed to assess the anatomy of the pelvic organs and the lower urinary tract. In patients with prior radiation, biopsy may be indicated to rule out recurrence of tumor.

Three types of vaginal reconstruction will be discussed: (1) the MacIndoe procedure using a partial thickness skin graft, (2) the use of gracilis muscle myocutaneous flaps, and (3) the use of bowel.

CREATION OF NEOVAGINA USING SKIN GRAFT

This procedure using skin grafts is probably the easiest and most successful method.

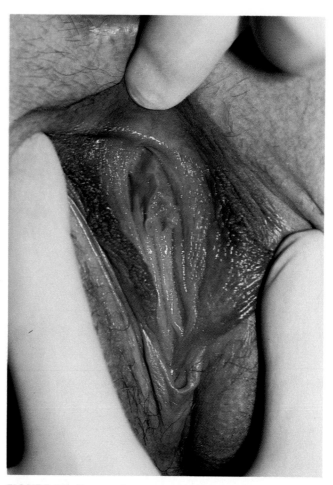

FIGURE 15–1. Vaginal examination of a patient with congenital absence of vagina.

SURGICAL TECHNIQUE

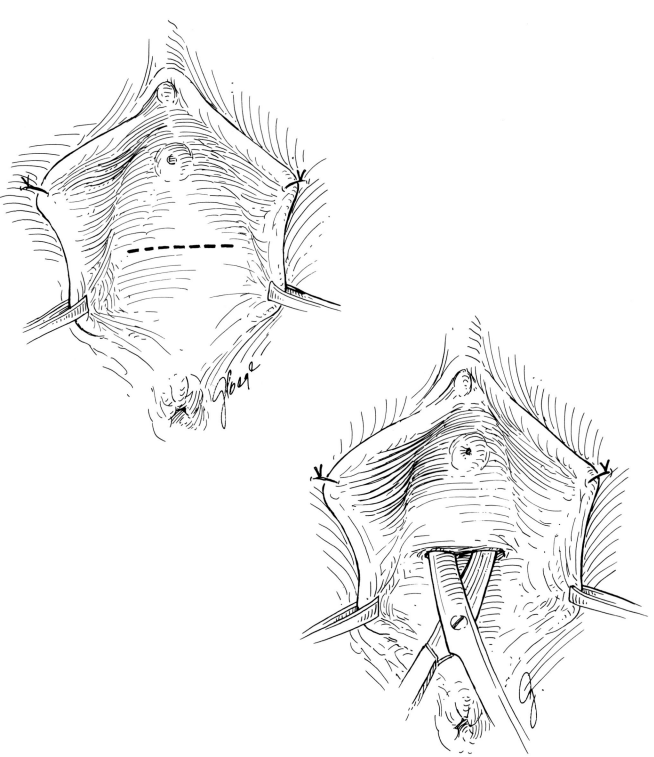

STEP 1:

After urethral catheterization, a transverse incision is made in the medial raphe between the urethra and anus. The incision allows for the formation of cutaneous flaps so that circumferential scar contraction can be avoided.

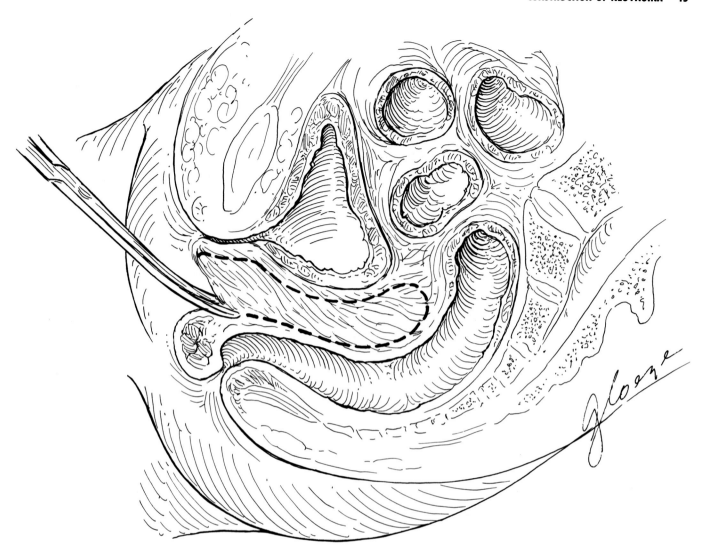

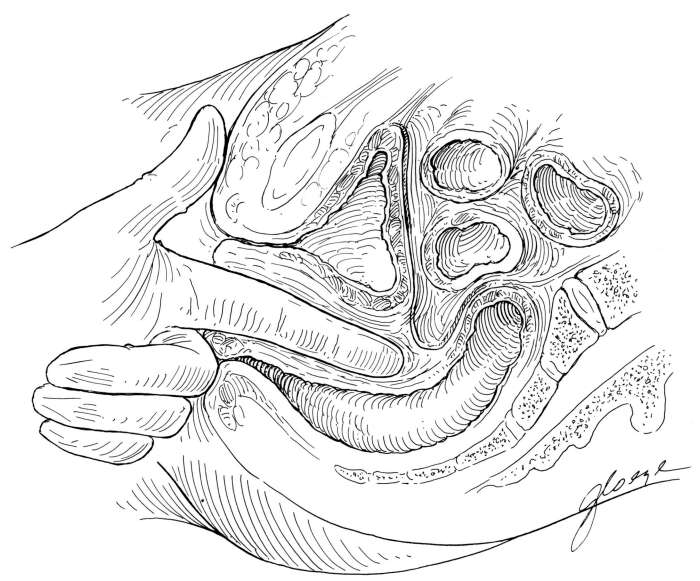

STEP 2:

The dissection is carried out sharply and bluntly in the space between bladder and rectum until the peritoneal fold is reached. The depth of the dissection should be exaggerated because of expected subsequent contraction; it should be in the range of 10 to 14 cm in an adult.

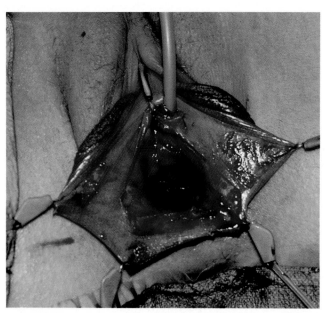

STEP 3:

The neovaginal canal is formed, separating rectum from bladder and urethra above the levator plate.

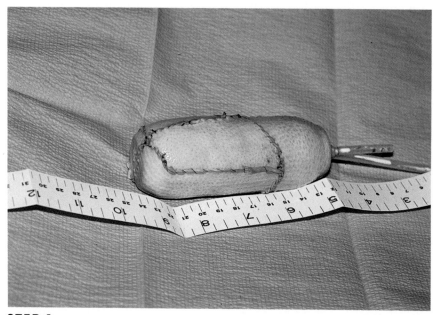

STEP 4:

Three split thickness skin graft sheets have been harvested from the buttock and hip area and reconfigured over a lubricated and partially inflated stent. Any dermatome can be used to obtain 2 to 3 sheets of skin for a total dimension of 14 × 7 cm. The length of the vaginal canal is measured, and an appropriate soft, pliable, inflatable stent is used. After inflation of the stent and proper lubrication of its outer surface, the skin graft sheets are sutured to each other and placed over the stent with the raw side out. The epidermal part of the skin faces the stent.

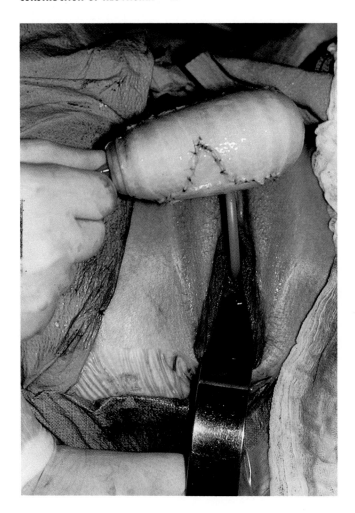

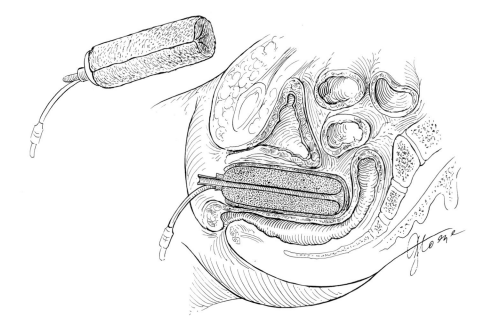

STEP 5:

The stent covered by the skin graft is ready to be inserted into the neovaginal canal as it is exposed with a posterior retractor. The end of the stent, covered by the skin graft, is seeded into the depth of the vaginal canal. The edges of the skin incision are sutured to the most superficial end of the skin graft. Interrupted silk sutures are used to fix the stent to the labia, ensuring that the stent will not slide out.

Postoperative Care and Complications

Postoperatively the patient remains in bed for a minimum of 5 days. After this period, the labial sutures are removed, the stent deflated, and the graft inspected. The stent can be washed and replaced immediately. This maneuver may be repeated as required. The conformer must be worn for a minimal period of 6 months. If this is not done, contraction of the vaginal canal will ensue. After 3 to 4 months, vaginal intercourse is allowed.

The most important complication of this procedure is vaginal stenosis due to contraction of the vaginal canal. Another skin flap may be required to enlarge further the vaginal canal. The skin has no secretory abilities, therefore patients require use of lubrication prior to intercourse. Rectal or urinary tract injury may occur during the dissection (a full lower bowel preparation should be done prior to surgery).

VAGINAL RECONSTRUCTION USING GRACILIS MUSCLE MYOCUTANEOUS FLAPS

The basic principles of this procedure are discussed in Chapter 7, on repair of vesicovaginal fistula. The gracilis myocutaneous flaps are used mainly after radiation injury and in reconstruction after extensive ablative surgery, such as anterior exenteration or total vaginectomy.

The vaginal canal is prepared as required with a length of at least 14 cm. With the patient in the lithotomy position, unilateral or bilateral island skin and gracilis muscle graft can be harvested. The flap can be tunneled under intact perineal skin and folded over the neovaginal canal. The donor site is closed in a linear fashion to reconstruct the vaginal depth. A conformer is not required after surgery.

VAGINAL RECONSTRUCTION USING BOWEL

In selected cases construction of a neovagina may be performed using bowel. Indications for surgery are mainly after failed skin graft or myocutaneous flap. Concomitant vaginectomy and bowel surgery make the use of a segment of bowel very appropriate. The sigmoid colon is commonly used because of its location and long pedicle, but other segments, like the cecum or flattened small bowel, can be used.

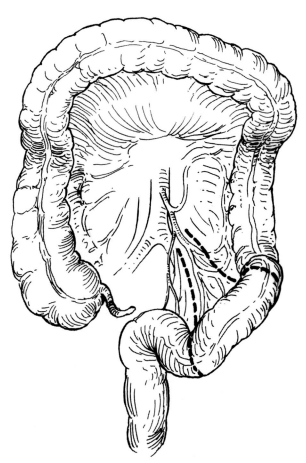

STEP 1:
Diagram of the colon and its sigmoid area. The neovaginal segment will be based on the inferior mesenteric artery.

STEP 2:
The patient is in the low lithotomy position. After preparation of the vaginal canal between rectum and bladder, the peritoneal fold is exposed. The abdomen is opened and explored for the most appropriate bowel segment to use, taking into consideration the length of the pedicle and its mobility. Using a combined vaginal and abdominal approach, the peritoneum at the cul de sac is opened, and a channel of sufficient width to transfer a segment of bowel is developed at the levator plate.

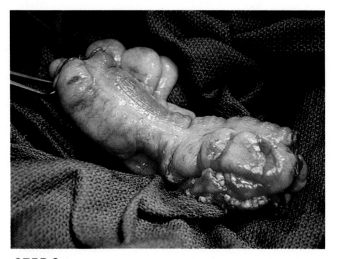

STEP 3:
A segment of 18 cm of sigmoid colon has been widely mobilized and isolated, using the gastrointestinal staple device.

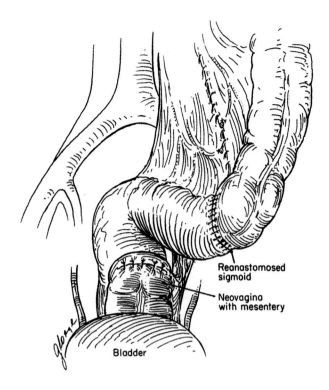

Reanastomosed
sigmoid

Neovagina
with mesentery

Bladder

STEP 4:

The colon has been reanastomosed and the neovaginal segment
advanced anterior to the colon toward the peritoneal cul de sac.

If the sigmoid colon is to be used, the peritoneum medial
and lateral to its mesothelium must be opened. The colon is
freed proximally and distally. Using a gastrointestinal stapler
device, a segment of colon 15 to 20 cm in length is isolated with
its vascular supply. The bowel is reanastomosed. The distal
segment of the free colonic tube is opened, the staples removed,
and the lumen irrigated with normal saline. The proximal line of
staples is reinforced with a running absorbable line of sutures.

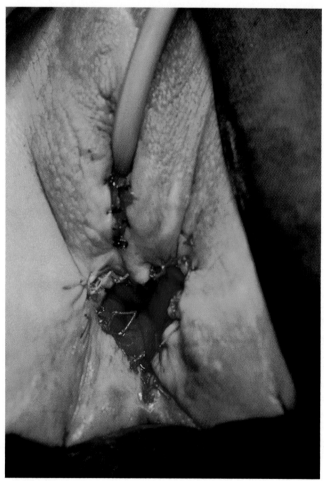

STEP 5:

The distal end of the bowel segment has been reanastomosed to
the introital skin.

The distal end of the neovaginal tube is transferred from
the abdominal to the vaginal area, making sure that no undue
tension is present in its pedicle. Interrupted sutures are used to
anastomose the vaginal introitus to the bowel segment.

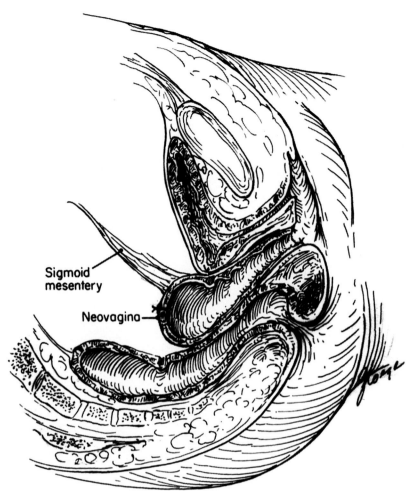

Sigmoid
mesentery

Neovagina

STEP 6:

Final view of the position of the bowel segment between the
rectum and bladder.

SIMPLE VULVECTOMY

FOR VULVAR

DYSTROPHY

INDICATIONS

This operation is very rarely performed in patients with severe benign disease, like vulvar dystrophy not responding to local treatment with testosterone cream or other local treatment (Fig. 16–1). The goal of surgery is to limit the excision to the vulvar skin without the need to perform a wide resection.

DIAGNOSIS

The clinical symptoms of severe vulvar dystrophy include severe pruritus; thin, shiny parchment skin; adhesions of the labia; stenosis; and destroyed architecture of the vulva. Carcinoma in situ should be ruled out. This condition is not related to estrogen deficiency; rather, testosterone is the treatment of choice. As mentioned, surgical therapy is rarely indicated.

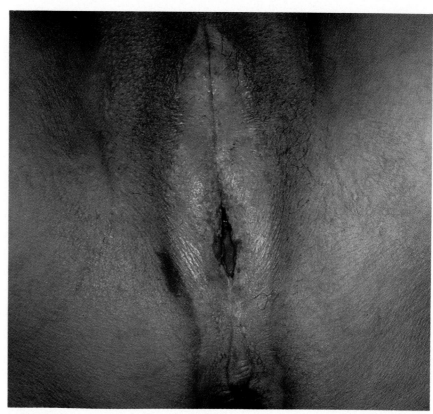

FIGURE 16–1. Severe symptoms of end-stage vulvar dystrophy not responding to therapy.

SURGICAL TECHNIQUE

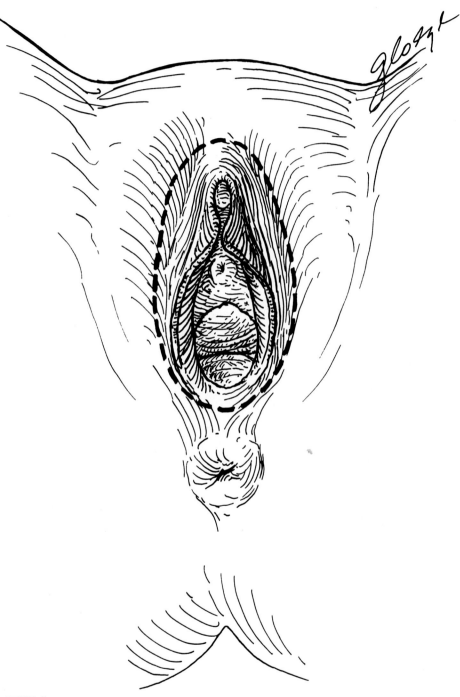

STEP 1:

With the patient in the lithotomy position, the vagina is prepared and draped. A Foley catheter is inserted into the bladder and a lubricated pack inserted into the rectum. An elliptical incision is made lateral to the labia majora, reaching superiorly the inferior rami of the symphysis and inferiorly the perineum before the rectum. The depth of the incision extends only to the subcutaneous fat. The use of a ring clamp with hooks will facilitate the exposure.

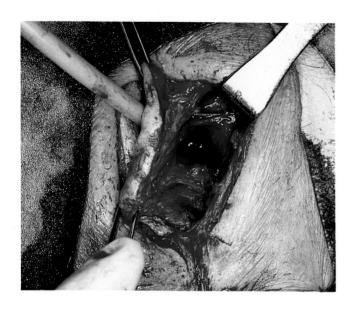

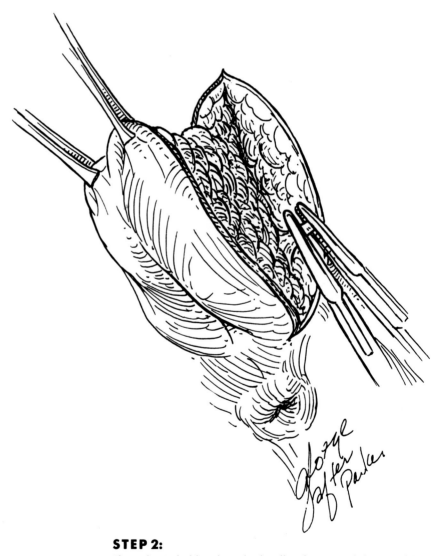

STEP 2:

The vulva is held with multiple Allis clamps and dissected free from the surrounding tissue.

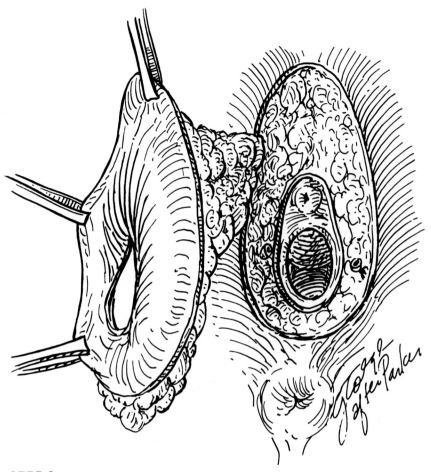

STEP 3:

A separate incision is made on the external margin of the vaginal canal as it joins the vulva. This second elliptical incision starts above the external urethral meatus and extends to the vaginal margins laterally and posteriorly. Care should be taken to avoid damage to the urethra or rectum.

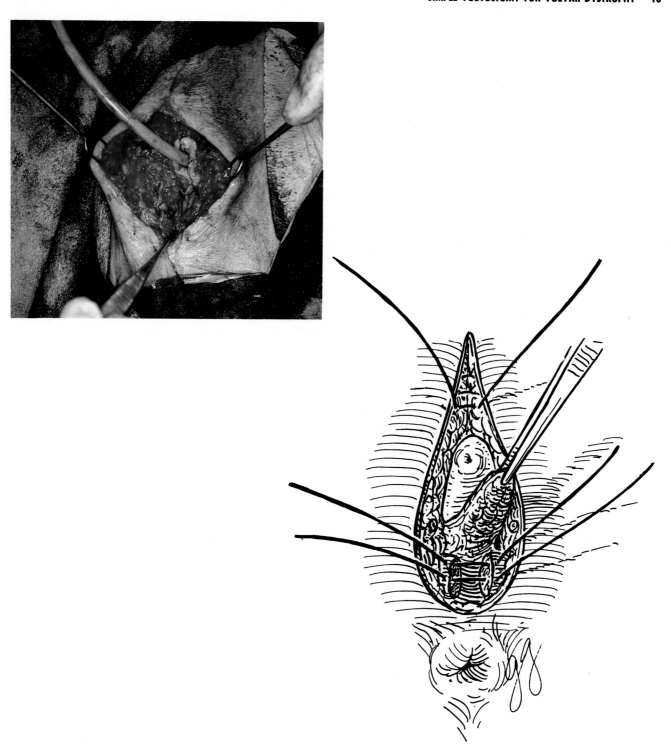

STEP 4:

The margins of the vaginal canal and urethra are exposed. The perineal skin is undermined and mobilized; proper hemostasis must be obtained. The skin in the mons pubis area is closed vertically. In the perineum, interrupted mattress sutures approximate the levator muscles. The skin is closed in a vertical fashion with two layers of subcutaneous and intradermic sutures. The suture line must be tension free. If required, further mobilization or a relaxing incision of the perineum should be made. An elliptical defect is created for the anastomosis of the perineal skin to the vagina.

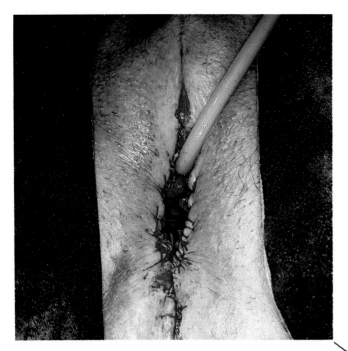

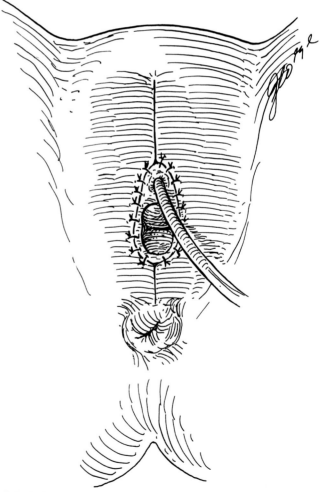

STEP 5:

After proper mobilization of its distal third, the vaginal canal is advanced. Interrupted absorbable sutures are used to anastomose the vagina to the perineal skin.

TRANSVAGINAL

DRAINAGE OF

PELVIC COLLECTION

Indications

When a collection of serum, pus, or blood is present in the cul de sac and drainage is indicated, the transvaginal route provides good access to the area. This approach will obviate the need for laparotomy, facilitating the post-operative recovery.

Diagnosis

Pelvic infection, irritative bladder symptoms, pelvic pain or pressure, rectal pain or dysfunction, and fever of unknown origin after operation may be symptoms of a pelvic collection. On physical examination, the cul de sac may be tender or distended. Ultrasound or computed tomography of the pelvis will delineate best the size and extent of the collection. A large ovarian cyst or a distended loop of bowel in the cul de sac may mimic a pelvic collection. The urinary tract should be evaluated to rule out urinoma. When pelvic ultrasound is done, a fine needle transvaginal aspiration may help in the diagnosis.

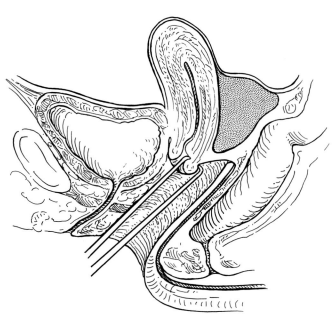

STEP 1:

The lower bowel should be prepared before surgery. The patient is in the lithotomy position, and after preparation and draping, the bladder is drained with a Foley catheter. A weighted speculum is inserted into the vagina, exposing the vaginal vault. If the uterus is present, a tenaculum is used to grasp the cervix and pull the cervix anteriorly. This maneuver will open the cul de sac.

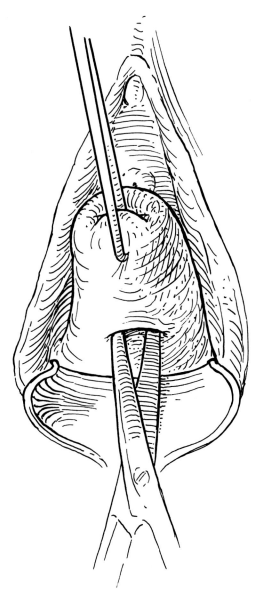

STEP 2:

A small needle is inserted into the cul de sac and the fluid aspirated. The depth and direction of the needle are noted. Transvaginal ultrasound may help in selecting the best area for drainage. A small incision is made behind the cervix or at the point of maximal bulge.

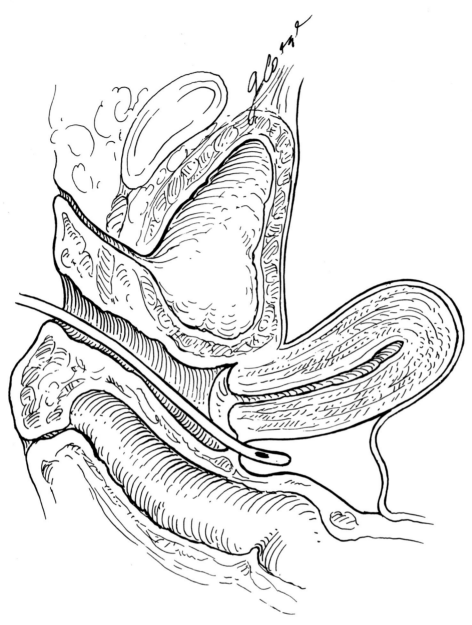

STEP 3:

Using blunt dissection, the cavity is entered and drained, and a small self-retaining catheter is inserted. Ultrasound should confirm the disappearance of the collection. The catheter may be removed in 2 days.

INDEX

Note: Page numbers in *italics* refer to illustrations.

ISBN 0-7216-2431-6

90071